LWW.com

Dedicated to:

. . . My husband *Bill*, my son *Brian*, and my daughter *Susan*, who all continue to support and encourage my academic pursuits.

MATH FOR NURSES

A Pocket Guide to Dosage Calculation and Drug Preparation

Mary Jo Boyer, RN, DNSc

Vice President, Chester County Operations
Adjunct Nursing Faculty and
  Former Dean and Professor of Nursing
  and Allied Health
Delaware County Community College
Media, Pennsylvania

7th *Edition*

 Wolters Kluwer | Lippincott Williams & Wilkins
Health

Philadelphia · Baltimore · New York · London
Buenos Aires · Hong Kong · Sydney · Tokyo

Senior Acquisitions Editor: Hilarie Surrena
Senior Managing Editor: Helen Kogut
Editorial Assistant: Elizabeth Harris
Production Project Manager: Cynthia Rudy
Director of Nursing Production: Helen Ewan
Senior Managing Editor / Production: Erika Kors
Design Coordinator: Joan Wendt
Manufacturing Coordinator: Karin Duffield
Production Services / Compositor: Aptara, Inc.

7th edition

9 8 7 6 5 4 3 2 1

Printed in China

Library of Congress Cataloging-in-Publication Data

Boyer, Mary Jo.
   Math for nurses : a pocket guide to dosage calculation and drug preparation / Mary Jo Boyer. — 7th ed.
      p. ; cm.
   Includes index.
   ISBN 978-0-7817-6335-6
   1. Nursing—Mathematics—Handbooks, manuals, etc. 2. Pharmaceutical arithmetic—Handbooks, manuals, etc. I. Title.
   [DNLM: 1. Pharmaceutical Preparations—administration & dosage—Handbooks. 2. Pharmaceutical Preparations—administration & dosage—Nurses' Instruction. 3. Dosage Forms—Handbooks. 4. Dosage Forms—Nurses' Instruction. 5. Mathematics—Handbooks. 6. Mathematics—Nurses' Instruction. QV 735 BL661m 2009]
   RT68.B68 2009
   615'.1401513—dc22

                                                          2008024064

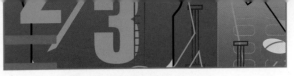

Contributors

Brian D. Boyer, AS, BA
Mathematics Instructor
Archdiocese of Philadelphia
Philadelphia, Pennsylvania

Elaine Dreisbaugh, BSN, MSN, CPN
Assistant Professor of Nursing
Delaware County Community College
Media, Pennsylvania
Former Nurse Educator, The Chester County Hospital
West Chester, Pennsylvania

Nancy J. Marquette, BSN, MSN, WOCN, CDE
Former Clinical Diabetic Nurse Educator
The Chester County Hospital
West Chester, Pennsylvania

Joanne O'Brian, BSN, MSN
Assistant Professor of Nursing
Delaware County Community College
Media, Pennsylvania
Nurse Educator, The Chester County Hospital
West Chester, Pennsylvania

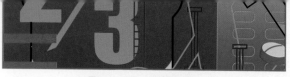

Reviewers

Jane Benedict, MSN, BSN
Associate Professor
Pennsylvania College of Technology
Williamsport, Pennsylvania

Dorothy Craig, RN, MSc
Instructor
Luzerne County Community College
Nanticoke, Pennsylvania

Nancy Harrer
Assistant Professor
Community College of Baltimore County
Catonsville, Maryland

Kelly Kidd
Nursing Coordinator
Algonquin College
Ottawa, Ontario

Caron Martin, MSN, RN
Associate Professor
Northern Kentucky University
Highland Heights, Kentucky

Dorothy Mathers, MSN
Associate Professor
Pennsylvania College of Technology
Williamsport, Pennsylvania

Dorothy Perri, RN, RNC, MS, BSN
ADN Instructor
Navarro College
Corsicana, Texas

Tami Rodgers, DVM, BSN
Professor of Nursing
Valencia Community College
Orlando, Florida

Alice Schmidt, MS
Professor
Ivy Tech Community College
Lafayette, Indiana

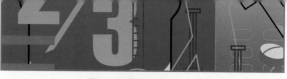

Preface

The idea for this compact, pocket-sized book about dosage calculation was generated by my students. For several years I watched as they took their math-related handouts and photocopied them, reducing them to a size that would fit into the pockets of their uniforms or laboratory coats. This "pocket" reference material was readily accessible when a math calculation was needed to administer a drug. Each year the number of papers that were copied increased as each group of students passed on their ideas to the next group. I also noted that staff nurses were using this readily available and compact information as a reference for math problems.

When a student then asked: "Why not put together for us all the information that we need?" I thought, "Why not?" The idea was born, the commit-ment made, and 18 months later the first edition of *Math for Nurses* was published in 1987. It is my hope that it will continue, in this seventh edition, to be help-ful to all who need a quick reference source when struggling with dosage calculations and drug preparation.

How to Use This Book

This book is designed for two purposes:

- To help you learn how to quickly and accurately calculate drug dosages and administer medications.
- To serve as a quick reference when reinforcement of learning is required.

The best way to use this pocket guide is to:

- Read the rules and examples.
- Follow the steps for solving the problems.
- Work the practice problems.
- Write down your answers and notes in the margin so that you have a quick reference when you need to review.

Organization

This pocket guide is divided into three units to facilitate quick access to specific information needed to administer drugs. The preassessment test should be completed before beginning. Unit 1 presents a review of basic math. Chapters 2 and 3 cover common fractions and decimals. Chapter 4 shows how to set up a ratio and proportion and solve for *x*, using a colon or fraction format. Drug-related word problems are used as contemporary examples. This unit information is essential, forming a foundation for understanding the complex dosage calculations presented in Unit 3.

Unit 2 explains measurement systems. The metric system, the apothecary system, and household units of measurement can be found in Chapters 5 and 6. Chapter 7 presents approximate system equivalents and shows how to convert from one unit of measurement to another. Some of these system equivalents are duplicated on the inside front cover of the book, to provide quick and easy access when calculating drug dosage problems.

Unit 3, Dosage Calculations, is the most comprehensive and detailed section of this pocket guide. The unit begins with a detailed description of how to read and interpret medication labels in chapter 8. Sample dosage questions specific to a drug label are used as examples. Chapters 9 and 10 cover oral and parenteral dosage problems. The Formula Method and Dimensional Analysis are introduced in Chapter 9. Critical care applications can be found in Chapter 12. Throughout this unit, problem-solving methodology is presented in a simple, easy-to-follow manner. A step-by-step approach is used, which will guide the reader through each set of examples. Enrichment information can be found in the appendices.

Special Features

A **pocket-size laminated card** containing approximate system equivalents and conversion formulas is included for quick and easy access when calculating drug dosage problems. This popular feature has been retained in this edition along with the Critical Thinking checks, questions designed to help you analyze the results of your answer to a dosage problem. They appear frequently throughout the book.

New Content in This Edition

- **Dimensional analysis (DA)** is presented in Chapter 9. Along with ratio and proportion and the Formula Method, DA is used throughout Chapters 9-15 as an example of an alternate way to solve dosage problems. Additional practice questions using DA are in every chapter and unit test.
- **Learning objectives** have been added to every chapter to help guide you in your learning.
- **New questions**—approximately 300—have been added throughout the book.

- **New appendix**—Appendix J, Nursing Considerations for Critical Care Drug Administration—alerts you to precautionary measures necessary in critical care.

Revised and Expanded Chapters

- Chapter 6: The Apothecary System and Household Equivalents
- Chapter 7: Approximate Equivalents and System Conversions
- Chapter 9: Oral Dosage Calculations
- Chapter 12: Intravenous Therapies: Critical Care Applications
- Chapter 13: Insulin
- Chapter 14: Heparin Preparation and Dosage Calculations
- Chapter 15: Pediatric Dosage Calculations and Intravenous Therapy

Math for Nurses was written for all nurses who administer drugs. It is intended as a quick, easy, and readily accessible guide when dosage calculations are required. It is my hope that its use will help nurses to calculate dosages accurately and, as a result, to improve the accuracy of drug delivery. As you use this book, please email me at mboyermboyer@dccc.edu with your comments and/or suggestions for improvement.

It is our inherent responsibility as nurses to ensure that every patient entrusted to our care receives the correct dosage of medication delivered in the most appropriate way.

Mary Jo Boyer, RN, DNSc

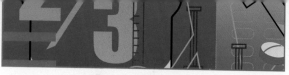

Contents

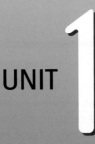

UNIT 1

Basic Mathematics Review and Refresher

This unit presents a basic review of fractions, decimals, percents, and ratio-proportion. The ability to solve for *x* assumes a basic mastery of fractions and decimals. Therefore, a brief review of addition, subtraction, multiplication, and division for fractions and decimals has been provided in Chapters 2 and 3 so you can review this material. In order to accurately calculate dosage problems, you need to be able to transcribe a word problem into a mathematical equation. This process is presented in a "step-by-step" format in Chapter 4. An end-of-unit review is provided for reinforcement of rules.

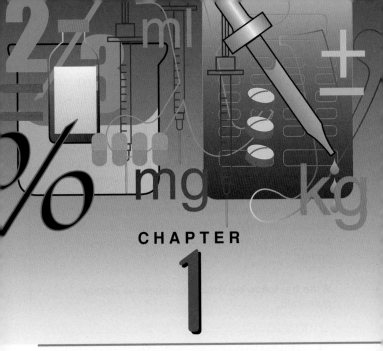

Preassessment Test: Mathematics Skills Review

Basic math skills are needed to calculate most dosage and solution problems encountered today in clinical practice. This pretest will help you understand your level of competence in solving fraction, decimal, and percentage problems as well as solving for the value of an unknown (*x*) using ratio-proportion.

The pretest has 16 sections comprising 100 questions, each worth one point. Answers are listed in the back of the book. A score of 90% or greater means that you have mastered the knowledge necessary to proceed directly to Unit II. Begin by setting aside 1 hour. You will need scrap paper. Take time to work out your answers and avoid careless mistakes. If an answer is incorrect, please review the corresponding section in Unit I. If you need to review Roman numerals and associated Arabic equivalents, please refer to Appendix A before beginning the pretest.

Write the following Arabic numbers as Roman numerals.

1. 8 _____   2. 13 _____

3. 2.5 _____   4. 37 _____

5. 51 _____

Write the following Roman numerals as Arabic numbers.

6. xi$\overline{\text{ss}}$ _____   7. xvi _____

8. LXV _____   9. ix _____

10. xix _____

Add or subtract the following fractions. Reduce to lowest terms.

11. $\dfrac{1}{2} + \dfrac{1}{8} =$ _____   12. $\dfrac{3}{4} - \dfrac{1}{4} =$ _____

13. $\dfrac{1}{5} + \dfrac{3}{10} =$ _____   14. $\dfrac{4}{6} - \dfrac{2}{5} =$ _____

Choose the fraction that has the largest value.

15. $\frac{1}{3}$ or $\frac{1}{6}$ _____

16. $\frac{1}{150}$ or $\frac{1}{200}$ _____

17. $\frac{1}{100}$ or $\frac{1}{150}$ _____

18. $\frac{1}{2}$ or $\frac{3}{4}$ _____

Multiply or divide the following fractions. Reduce to lowest terms.

19. $\frac{1}{2} \times \frac{3}{4} =$ _____

20. $2\frac{2}{5} \times 3\frac{5}{10} =$ _____

21. $\frac{1}{4} \div \frac{1}{3} =$ _____

22. $3\frac{1}{2} \div \frac{4}{7} =$ _____

23. $\frac{1}{150} \times 2\frac{1}{2} =$ _____

24. $\frac{8}{7} \times 3 =$ _____

25. $\frac{1}{8} \div 6 =$ _____

26. $4\frac{2}{5} \div 11 =$ _____

Change the following mixed numbers to improper fractions.

27. $2\frac{4}{5}$ _____

28. $6\frac{3}{4}$ _____

29. $10\frac{4}{9}$ _____

30. $8\frac{1}{7}$ _____

Reduce these improper fractions to whole or mixed numbers. Reduce to lowest terms.

31. $\frac{120}{40}$ _____

32. $\frac{146}{36}$ _____

33. $\dfrac{35}{11}$ _____   34. $\dfrac{16}{13}$ _____

Change the following fractions to decimals.
Remember to place a "0" before the decimal point
when the decimal is less than (<) one.

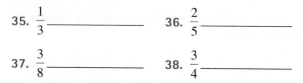

35. $\dfrac{1}{3}$ _____   36. $\dfrac{2}{5}$ _____

37. $\dfrac{3}{8}$ _____   38. $\dfrac{3}{4}$ _____

Add or subtract the following decimals.

39. $0.36 + 1.45 =$ _____

40. $3.71 + 0.29 =$ _____

41. $6 - 0.13 =$ _____

42. $2.14 - 0.01 =$ _____

Multiply or divide the following decimals.

43. $6 \times 8.13 =$ _____

44. $0.125 \times 2 =$ _____

45. $21.6 \div 0.3 =$ _____

46. $7.82 \div 2.3 =$ _____

Change the following decimals to fractions. Reduce
to lowest terms.

47. 0.25 _____   48. 0.80 _____

49. 0.33 _____   **50.** 0.45 _____

51. 0.75 _____   **52.** 0.60 _____

Solve for the value of x in the following ratio and proportion problems.

53. $4.2 : 14 :: x : 10$ _____

54. $0.8 : 4 :: 3.2 : x$ _____

55. $6 : 2 :: 8 : x$ _____

56. $5 : 20 :: x : 40$ _____

57. $0.25 : 200 :: x : 600$ _____

58. $\dfrac{1}{5} : x :: \dfrac{1}{20} : 3$ _____

59. $12 : x :: 8 : 16$ _____

60. $x : \dfrac{4}{5} :: 0.60 : 3$ _____

61. $0.3 : 12 :: x : 36$ _____

62. $x : 8 :: \dfrac{1}{4} : 10$ _____

Change the following fractions and decimals to percentages.

63. $\dfrac{1}{5}$ _____   **64.** 0.36 _____

65. 0.07 _____   **66.** $\dfrac{5}{40}$ _____

67. 0.103 _____   **68.** 1.83 _____

69. $\dfrac{4}{16}$ _____ **70.** 60/100 _____

71. 0.01 _____ **72.** 1.98 _____

73. $\dfrac{120}{100}$ _____ **74.** $\dfrac{8}{56}$ _____

Change the following percents to decimals.

75. 25% _____ **76.** 40% _____

77. 80% _____ **78.** 15% _____

79. 4.8% _____ **80.** 0.36% _____

81. 1.75% _____ **82.** 8.30% _____

Solve the following percent equations.

83. 30% of 60 _____

84. 4.5% of 200 _____

85. 0.6% of 180 _____

86. 30 is 75% of _____

87. 20 is 80% of _____

88. What % of 80 is 20 _____

89. What % of 60 is 12 _____

90. What % of 72 is 18 _____

91. 15 is 30% of _____

92. 60 is 50% of _____

Write each of the following measures in its related equivalency. Reduce to lowest terms.

	Percent	Ratio	Common Fraction	Decimal
93.	25%	_____	_____	_____
94.	_____	1 : 30	_____	_____
95.	_____	_____	_____	0.05
96.	_____	_____	$\frac{1}{150}$	_____
97.	0.45%	_____	_____	_____
98.	_____	1 : 100	_____	_____
99.	_____	_____	$\frac{1}{120}$	_____
100.	_____	_____	_____	0.50

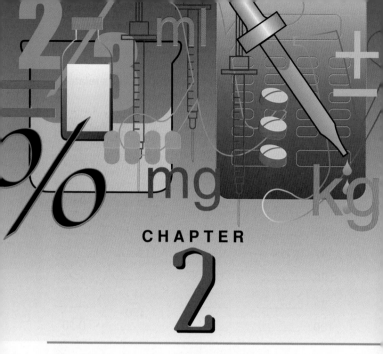

2

Common Fractions

LEARNING OBJECTIVES

After completing this chapter, you should be able to:

- Understand the concept of a fraction, the number of parts to a whole.
- Distinguish between the four types of fractions, concept of size, and fraction value relative to the value of one (1).
- Convert fractions and reduce them to their lowest terms.
- Add, subtract, multiply, and divide fractions.

The term *fraction* means a type of division.
A *fraction* is a part or piece of a whole that *indicates
division of that whole into equal units or parts.*
Fractions are referred to as *common fractions,* which
are simply fractions as you recognize them (1/2, 1/3),
or *decimal fractions* (0.5, 0.33), which will be covered in Chapter 3. A fraction is written with one number over another, i.e., 1/4, 2/5; therefore, consider the
line between the numbers a *division sign.* The number
on *top of the line (numerator)* is divided by the number *under the line (denominator).* Because the fraction (1/4) represents division, it can be read as numerator (1) divided by denominator (4). You need to
know how to calculate dosage problems with fractions because they are used in apothecary and household measures as well as a variety of reports, medical
orders, and documents used in health care.

Look at the circles in Figure 2.1. They are
divided into equal parts (4 and 8). Each part of
the circle (1) is a fraction or piece of the whole
(1/4 or 1/8).

The Denominator of a Fraction

The denominator of a fraction tells you the total
number of equal parts into which the whole has been
divided. If you divide a circle into four equal parts,
the *total number of parts* (4) that you are working
with is the *bottom* number of the fraction and is
called the *denominator.* If you divide the circle into
eight equal parts, the denominator is 8. The denominator can also be called the *divisor.*

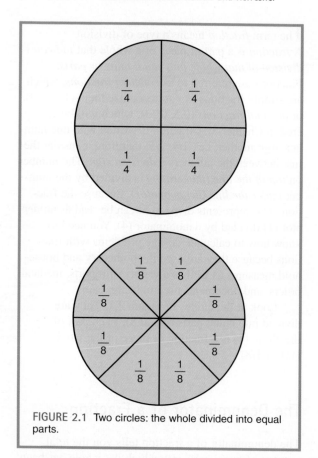

FIGURE 2.1 Two circles: the whole divided into equal parts.

RULE: The denominator refers to the *total number of equal parts* and is the number on the bottom of the fraction. The larger the number in the denominator, the smaller the value of the equal parts (or fraction) of the whole. See Figure 2.1.

The Numerator of a Fraction

The numerator of a fraction tells you how many parts of the whole are being considered. If you divide a circle into four equal parts, each part (1) that you are considering is the *top* number of the fraction and is called the *numerator*. If you divide the circle into eight equal parts, and you are considering three parts, the numerator is three (3). The numerator can also be called the *dividend*.

> **RULE:** The numerator refers to *a part* of the whole that is being considered and is the number on the top of the fraction. The larger the number in the numerator, the more parts of the whole that are being considered. For the fraction 3/8, three parts of the total (8) are being considered.

Using the circle examples in Figure 2.1, the numerator in both is 1 and the denominator is either 4 or 8.

$$\text{Fraction} = \frac{1}{4} \text{ or } \frac{1}{8} = \frac{\text{numerator}}{\text{denominator}} = \text{"divided by"}$$

PRACTICE PROBLEMS

Use the first problem as an example. Fill in the blanks for the rest.

1. 7/8 means that you have _7_ equal parts, each worth 1/8. The numerator is _7_ divided by the denominator, which is _8_.

2. 9/10 means that you have _____ equal parts, each worth _____. The denominator is _____.

3. 4/5 means that you have _____ equal parts, each worth _____. The numerator is _____ divided by the denominator, which is _____.

4. 3/4 means that you have _____ equal parts, each worth _____. The denominator is _____.

Concept of Size

> **RULE: When the numerators are the same, the larger the number in the denominator, the *smaller the value of the parts* (or fraction) of the whole.**

Look at Figure 2.1, which illustrates two circles: one is divided into fourths, and one is divided into eighths. As you look at the circles, you will notice that the circle that is divided into eighths has smaller portions than the circle that is divided into fourths. The reason is that the value of each part of the fraction 1/8 is less than the value of each part of the fraction 1/4. Even though 1/8 has a larger denominator (8) than does 1/4 (4), it is a smaller fraction. This is an important concept to understand; that is, the larger the number or value in the denominator, the smaller the fraction or parts of the whole. For example:

$$\frac{1}{2} \text{ is larger than } \frac{1}{4}$$

$$\frac{1}{8} \text{ is larger than } \frac{1}{16}$$

$$\frac{1}{9} \text{ is larger than } \frac{1}{10}$$

RULE: When the denominators are the same, the larger the number in the numerator, the *larger the value of the parts* of the whole.

Look at Figure 2.2. The shaded area in the top circle shows that 3/4 is larger than 1/4. The shaded area in the bottom circle shows that 5/8 is larger than 3/8.

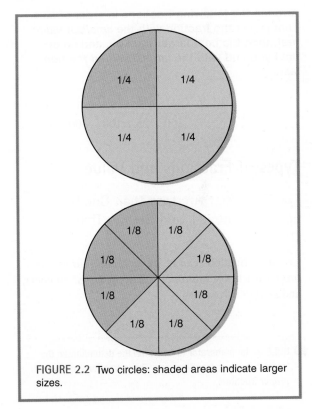

FIGURE 2.2 Two circles: shaded areas indicate larger sizes.

PRACTICE PROBLEMS

Indicate which fractions are larger.

1. 1/2 or 1/4 _____   2. 1/8 or 1/16 _____

3. 1/9 or 1/10 _____   4. 2/5 or 4/5 _____

5. 1/6 or 4/6 _____   6. 3/15 or 8/15 _____

Arrange the following fractions in order of size.
That is, list the fraction with the *smallest value*
first, then the next larger fraction, and so on
until you end with the *largest valued fraction*
last.

$$\frac{1}{9} \quad \frac{1}{12} \quad \frac{1}{3} \quad \frac{1}{7} \quad \frac{1}{150} \quad \frac{1}{25} \quad \frac{1}{100} \quad \frac{1}{300} \quad \frac{1}{75}$$

Types of Fractions and Value

Fractions That Are Less Than One (<1), Equal to One (1), and Greater Than One (>1)

Common fractions can be divided into four groups:
proper fractions, *improper* fractions, *mixed numbers,*
and *complex fractions.*

> **RULE:** If the numerator is *less than* the denominator, the
> fraction value is *less than one.* These fractions are called
> *proper* fractions.

Examples: $\dfrac{3}{4} < 1,$ $\dfrac{7}{8} < 1,$ $\dfrac{9}{10} < 1$

RULE: If the numerator and denominator are *equal to each other,* the fraction value is *equal to one.* These fractions are called *improper* fractions.

Examples: $\dfrac{1}{1} = 1,$ $\dfrac{3}{3} = 1,$ $\dfrac{25}{25} = 1$

RULE: If the numerator is *greater than* the denominator, the fraction value is *greater than one.* These fractions are also called *improper* fractions.

Examples: $\dfrac{2}{1} = 2 > 1,$ $\dfrac{5}{4} = 1\dfrac{1}{4} > 1$

RULE: If a fraction and a whole number are *written together,* the fraction value is *always greater than one.* These fractions are *mixed* numbers.

Examples: $1\dfrac{1}{2} > 1,$ $3\dfrac{3}{4} > 1,$ $5\dfrac{4}{5} > 1$

RULE: If a fraction includes a combination of whole numbers and proper and improper fractions in both the numerator and the denominator, the value may be *less than, equal to,* or *greater than one.* These fractions are called *complex* fractions.

Examples: $\dfrac{\dfrac{1}{2}}{2} < 1 \qquad \dfrac{\dfrac{3}{12}}{\dfrac{5}{20}} = 1 \qquad \dfrac{\dfrac{8}{14}}{\dfrac{1}{3}} > 1$

Equivalent or Equal Fractions

Changing Fractions to Equivalent or Equal Fractions

When you are working problems with fractions, it is sometimes necessary to change a fraction to a different but equivalent fraction to make the math problem easier to calculate. For example, it may be necessary to change 2/4 to 1/2 or 2/3 to 4/6. You can make a new fraction that has the same value by either multiplying or dividing *both the numerator and the denominator by the same number.* Look at the following examples.

Examples: $\dfrac{2}{3}$ can be changed to $\dfrac{4}{6}$ by multiplying both the numerator and the denominator by 2.

$$\left(\dfrac{2 \times 2 = 4}{3 \times 2 = 6} \right)$$

$\dfrac{2}{4}$ can be changed to $\dfrac{1}{2}$ by dividing both the numerator and the denominator by 2.

$$\left(\dfrac{2 \div 2 = 1}{4 \div 2 = 2} \right)$$

It is important to remember that you can change the numerator and the denominator of a fraction and the value of the fraction will be unchanged *as long as you follow the following rule:*

> RULE: When changing a fraction, yet keeping the same equivalent value, you must do the same thing (multiply or divide by the same number) to the numerator and to the denominator.

Examples: To change the fraction $\frac{4}{5}$ to $\frac{8}{10}$, multiply 4×2 and 5×2.

$$\left(\frac{4 \times 2 = 8}{5 \times 2 = 10} \right)$$

$\frac{4}{5}$ has the same value as $\frac{8}{10}$.

To change the fraction $\frac{4}{16}$ to $\frac{1}{4}$, divide 4 by 4 and 16 by 4.

$$\left(\frac{4 \div 4 = 1}{16 \div 4 = 4} \right)$$

To determine that both fractions have equal value, multiply the opposite numerators and denominators. For example, if 4/5 = 8/10, then the product of 4×10 will equal the product of 5×8.

$$4 \times 10 = 40 \quad \text{and} \quad 5 \times 8 = 40$$

PRACTICE PROBLEMS

Circle the correct answer.

1. 3/5 is equivalent to: 6/15 or 9/10 or 12/20

2. 4/8 is equivalent to: 8/24 or 12/16 or 20/40

3. 6/12 is equivalent to: 2/4 or 3/5 or 12/36

4. 10/16 is equivalent to: 20/48 or 5/8 or 30/32

5. 12/20 is equivalent to: 3/5 or 6/5 or 4/10

6. 18/30 is equivalent to: 3/15 or 9/10 or 6/10

7. 9/54 is equivalent to: 3/16 or 1/6 or 1/8

8. 15/90 is equivalent to: 1/6 or 3/8 or 5/14

9. 14/56 is equivalent to: 2/6 or 1/4 or 7/8

10. 8/144 is equivalent to: 2/36 or 4/23 or 1/18

Simplifying, or Reducing, Fractions to Lowest Terms

When calculating dosages, it is easier to work with fractions that have been simplified, or reduced to the lowest terms. This means that the numerator and the denominator are the smallest numbers that can still represent the fraction or piece of the whole. For example, 4/10 can be reduced to 2/5; 4/8 can be reduced to 1/2. It is important to know how to reduce (or simplify) a fraction. The following rule outlines the steps for reducing a fraction to its lowest terms. Remember: You may have to reduce several times.

> **RULE:** To reduce a fraction to its lowest terms: divide both the numerator and the denominator by the *largest* number that can go evenly into both.

Examples: Reduce the fraction $\dfrac{9}{18}$ to its lowest terms.

$$\left(\frac{9}{18} \begin{array}{c} \div\ 9\ =\ \dfrac{1}{2} \\ \div\ 9 \end{array} \right)$$

The largest number that can be used to divide *both* the numerator (9) and the denominator (18) is 9.

Reduce: $\dfrac{6}{10}$ can be reduced to $\dfrac{3}{5}$ by dividing both the numerator and the denominator by 2.

Reduce: $\dfrac{33}{132}$ can be reduced to $\dfrac{11}{44}$ by dividing both the numerator and the denominator by 3. Then $\dfrac{11}{44}$ can be reduced again to 1/4 by dividing by 11.

PRACTICE PROBLEMS

Reduce the following fractions to their lowest terms:

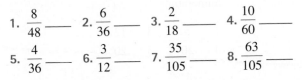

1. $\dfrac{8}{48}$ ____ 2. $\dfrac{6}{36}$ ____ 3. $\dfrac{2}{18}$ ____ 4. $\dfrac{10}{60}$ ____

5. $\dfrac{4}{36}$ ____ 6. $\dfrac{3}{12}$ ____ 7. $\dfrac{35}{105}$ ____ 8. $\dfrac{63}{105}$ ____

Finding the Least Common Denominator (LCD)

> **RULE: To find the least common denominator: find the** *smallest* **number that is easily divided by both denominators, and then change the fraction to equivalent fractions, each with the same denominator. Remember: least common denominator = smallest number.**

When beginning, first see if any of the denominators can be easily divided by each of the other denominators. If so, that number now becomes your new LCD.

Example: Add $\dfrac{1}{4} + \dfrac{3}{5}$

- Find the *smallest* number (LCD) that all the denominators can be divided evenly into.

$$\frac{1}{4} + \frac{3}{5} \qquad \text{The LCD} = 20$$

- Change the unlike fractions to equivalent or equal fractions using the LCD. Divide the LCD by the denominator and then multiply that number by the numerator.

$$\frac{1}{4} = \frac{5}{20} \qquad \frac{3}{5} = \frac{12}{20}$$

• Add the new numerators and place that number over the new LCD.

$$\frac{5}{20} + \frac{12}{20} = \frac{17}{20}$$

Answer: $\frac{17}{20}$

• Reduce and change any improper fraction to a mixed number, if necessary.

Example: Add $\frac{1}{3} + \frac{5}{6}$ The LCD = 6

• Change $\frac{1}{3}$ to $\frac{2}{6}$ and $\frac{5}{6}$ stays $\frac{5}{6}$

• Add the new numerators and place that number over the new LCD.

$$2 + 5 = 7 \quad \frac{7}{6}$$

• Change the improper fraction to a mixed number.

$\frac{7}{6}$ is changed to $1\frac{1}{6}$

Answer: $1\frac{1}{6}$

Conversion

Converting Mixed Numbers and Improper Fractions

You need to know how to convert a variety of fractions to make drug dosage calculations easier. Mixed numbers (1 1/4) can be changed to improper fractions (5/4) and improper fractions (3/2) can be changed to mixed numbers (1 1/2). If you get a final answer that is an improper fraction, convert it to a mixed number. For example, it is better to say "I have 1 1/4 apples" than to say "I have 5/4 apples."

To understand how to convert fractions, follow these rules.

Changing a Mixed Number to an Improper Fraction

> **RULE: To change a mixed number to an improper fraction: multiply the denominator by the whole number and then add the numerator to that sum.**

Example: Change $2\dfrac{3}{4}$ to an improper fraction.

$$2\frac{3}{4} = 4 \times 2 = 8 \qquad 8 + 3 = 11$$

The answer (11) becomes the *new numerator* of the new single fraction. The denominator in the original stays the same.

$$2\frac{3}{4} = \frac{11}{4}$$

The *mixed number* $2\frac{3}{4}$ becomes the *improper fraction* $\frac{11}{4}$.

PRACTICE PROBLEMS

Change the following mixed numbers to improper fractions:

1. $5\frac{9}{12}$ _____

2. $6\frac{7}{8}$ _____

3. $8\frac{3}{5}$ _____

4. $15\frac{1}{9}$ _____

5. $32\frac{2}{3}$ _____

6. $21\frac{3}{4}$ _____

7. $18\frac{1}{2}$ _____

8. $6\frac{3}{9}$ _____

9. $5\frac{2}{5}$ _____

10. $11\frac{1}{6}$ _____

Changing an Improper Fraction to a Mixed Number

RULE: To change an improper fraction to a mixed or whole number: divide the numerator by the denominator and then use the leftover numbers as the new numerator and the new denominator of the mixed number. The quotient becomes the whole number of the mixed number.

Example: Change $\dfrac{13}{7}$ to a mixed number.

The number that you get (1) when you divide the numerator (13) by the denominator (7) becomes the whole number of the mixed number.

$13 \div 7 = 1$ (new whole number)

The *remainder,* or number that you have left over (6), becomes the numerator of the fraction that goes with the whole number to make it a mixed number.

$13 \div 7 = 1\dfrac{6}{?}$

The *original* denominator of the improper fraction (7) becomes the denominator of the fraction of the mixed number.

$13 \div 7 = 1\dfrac{6}{7}$

Any remainder is reduced to the lowest terms.

Answer: $1\dfrac{6}{7}$

PRACTICE PROBLEMS

Change the following improper fractions to mixed numbers:

1. $\dfrac{30}{4}$ _____

2. $\dfrac{41}{6}$ _____

3. $\dfrac{68}{9}$ _____   4. $\dfrac{72}{11}$ _____

5. $\dfrac{90}{12}$ _____   6. $\dfrac{40}{15}$ _____

7. $\dfrac{86}{20}$ _____   8. $\dfrac{62}{8}$ _____

9. $\dfrac{86}{9}$ _____   10. $\dfrac{112}{6}$ _____

Addition of Fractions

When fractions are added, *no calculations are done on the denominators.* Therefore, fractions can be added *only when the denominators are the same.* When adding fractions, *only the numerators are added!* Denominators that are different (unlike) must be made the same.

Addition of Fractions When the Denominators Are the Same

> **RULE: To add fractions with the same denominators: add the numerators and place the new sum over the similar denominator. Reduce to lowest terms and change to a mixed number if necessary.**

Example: Add $\dfrac{1}{5} + \dfrac{3}{5}$

- Add the numerators. For example:

$$\dfrac{1}{5} + \dfrac{3}{5} = \dfrac{1 + 3}{5} = 4$$

- Place the new sum over the same denominator.

$$\frac{1}{5} + \frac{3}{5} = \frac{4}{5} = \begin{array}{l} \text{new numerator} \\ \text{same denominator} \end{array}$$

Answer: $\frac{4}{5}$

Example: Add $\frac{1}{7} + \frac{4}{7}$

Change: $\frac{1}{7} + \frac{4}{7} = \frac{1+4}{7} = \frac{5}{7}$

$$\frac{5}{7} = \begin{array}{l} \text{new numerator} \\ \text{same denominaotor} \end{array}$$

Answer: $\frac{5}{7}$

Example: Add $\frac{1}{6} + \frac{9}{6}$

Change: $\frac{1}{6} + \frac{9}{6} = \frac{1+9}{6} = \frac{10}{6}$

$$\frac{10}{6} = \begin{array}{l} \text{new numerator} \\ \text{same denominaotor} \end{array}$$

$\frac{10}{6}$ needs to be reduced

Reduce: $\frac{10}{6} = \frac{10 \div 2}{6 \div 2} = \frac{5}{3} =$ improper fraction

Change: $\dfrac{5}{3} = 5 \div 3 = 1\dfrac{2}{3} = $ a mixed number

Answer: $1\dfrac{2}{3}$

Addition of Fractions When the Denominators Are Not the Same

> **RULE: To add fractions when the denominators are not the same: find the least common denominator of each fraction, take each new quotient and multiply it by each numerator, add the numerators, place the new sum over the LCD, and reduce to lowest terms.**

Example: Add $\dfrac{1}{4} + \dfrac{3}{5}$ The LCD is 20

- Divide the LCD of 20 by the denominator of each fraction to get the new *quotient*.

$$\dfrac{1}{4} = \dfrac{}{20} \qquad 20 \div 4 = 5$$

$$\dfrac{3}{5} = \dfrac{}{20} \qquad 20 \div 5 = 4$$

- Take each new quotient and multiply it by the numerator of each fraction.

$$5 \text{ (new quotient)} \times 1 \text{ (numerator)} = \dfrac{5}{20}$$

$$4 \text{ (new quotient)} \times 3 \text{ (numerator)} = \dfrac{12}{20}$$

• Add the new numerators. Place the new sum over the LCD. Reduce to lowest terms.

$$\frac{5}{20} + \frac{12}{20} = \frac{17}{20}$$

Answer: $\frac{17}{20}$

Example: Add $\frac{1}{3} + \frac{5}{6}$

• The least common denominator would be 6.

Change $\frac{1}{3}$ to $\frac{2}{6}$

Change $\frac{5}{6}$ to $\frac{5}{6}$

• Add the new numerators.

$$\frac{2}{6} + \frac{5}{6} = \frac{2+5}{6} = \frac{7}{6}$$

• Change any improper fraction to a mixed number.

$\frac{7}{6}$ should be changed to $1\frac{1}{6}$.

Answer: $1\frac{1}{6}$

Addition of Mixed Numbers

> **RULE: To add fractions with a mixed number: change any mixed number to an improper fraction, find the LCD, change to similar fractions, add the new numerators, and reduce to lowest terms.**

Example: Add $\dfrac{1}{6} + 2\dfrac{3}{8} + \dfrac{5}{6}$

- Change the mixed number to an improper fraction.

$$2\dfrac{3}{8} \text{ becomes } \dfrac{19}{8}$$

- Find the LCD. For the denominators of 6 and 8, use the LCD of 24.

- Change the different fractions to fractions with the same denominator.

$$\dfrac{1}{6} \text{ becomes } \dfrac{4}{24}$$

$$\dfrac{19}{8} \text{ becomes } \dfrac{57}{24}$$

$$\dfrac{5}{6} \text{ becomes } \dfrac{20}{24}$$

- Add the new numerators and place your answer over the LCD.

$$\dfrac{4 + 57 + 20}{} = \dfrac{81}{24}$$

- Reduce to lowest terms and change to a mixed number.

$$\frac{81}{24} = \frac{27}{8} = 3\frac{3}{8}$$

Answer: $3\dfrac{3}{8}$

Subtraction of Fractions

Fractions can be subtracted *only when the denominators are the same* because only the numerators are subtracted. Denominators that are unlike must be made the same.

Subtraction of Fractions When the Denominators Are the Same

> **RULE:** To subtract fractions when the denominators are the same, *only subtract the numerators.* Reduce to lowest terms.

To subtract fractions when the denominators are the same, simply subtract the numerators. To subtract 3/8 from 7/8, subtract 3 from 7, which equals 4. Place the new numerator (4) over the new denominator (8) and reduce to lowest terms (4/8 = 1/2).

Example: Subtract $\dfrac{5}{6} - \dfrac{3}{6}$

- Subtract $\dfrac{5}{6} - \dfrac{3}{6} = \dfrac{5 - 3}{6} = \dfrac{2}{6}$

- Reduce $\dfrac{2}{6} = \dfrac{1}{3}$, a new fraction

Answer: $\dfrac{1}{3}$

Example: Subtract $\dfrac{7}{8} - \dfrac{4}{8} = \dfrac{7-4}{} = \dfrac{3}{8}$

$\dfrac{3}{8}$, a new fraction

Answer: $\dfrac{3}{8}$

Example: Subtract $\dfrac{3}{8} - \dfrac{7}{8} = \dfrac{4}{8}$

- Reduce $\dfrac{4}{8} = \dfrac{1}{2}$, a new fraction

Answer: $\dfrac{1}{2}$

Subtraction of Fractions When the Denominators Are Not the Same

You will probably never need to subtract fractions with different denominators or fractions with a mixed number to calculate dosage problems. However, both will be presented here briefly just in case the situation occurs.

> **RULE: To subtract fractions when the denominators are not the same: find the LCD, change to similar fractions, and subtract the new numerators. Reduce to lowest terms.**

Example: Subtract $\dfrac{5}{6} - \dfrac{3}{5}$

- Find the least common denominator.

$$\dfrac{5}{6} - \dfrac{3}{5} = 30 \text{ (LCD)}$$

- Change to similar or equal fractions. Refer back to pages 22–28.

$$\dfrac{5}{6} \text{ becomes } \dfrac{25}{30}$$

$$\dfrac{3}{5} \text{ becomes } \dfrac{18}{30}$$

- Subtract the new numerators and place your answer over the common denominator:

$$\dfrac{25}{30} - \dfrac{18}{30} = \dfrac{25 - 18}{30} = \dfrac{7}{30}$$

Answer: $\dfrac{7}{30}$

Subtraction of Mixed Numbers

There are two ways to subtract fractions with mixed numbers:

Change the mixed number to an improper fraction or leave the mixed numbers as mixed numbers.

> **RULE: To subtract fractions with a mixed number: change the mixed number to an improper fraction, find the LCD, change to similar fractions, subtract the new numerators, and reduce to lowest terms.**

Example: Subtract $2\dfrac{1}{8} - \dfrac{3}{6}$

$$2\dfrac{1}{8} = \dfrac{17}{8} - \dfrac{3}{6}$$

- Find the LCD. For the denominators 8 and 6, use the LCD of 24.

- Change to similar or equal fractions.

$$\dfrac{17}{8} \text{ becomes } \dfrac{51}{24}$$

$$\dfrac{3}{6} \text{ becomes } \dfrac{12}{24}$$

- Subtract the new numerators and place your answer over the common denominator:

$$\dfrac{51}{24} - \dfrac{12}{24} = \dfrac{51-12}{24} = \dfrac{39}{24}$$

- Reduce and change to a mixed number, if necessary.

$$\dfrac{39}{24} \text{ becomes } \dfrac{13}{8} = 1\dfrac{5}{8}$$

Answer: $1\dfrac{5}{8}$

> **RULE: To subtract fractions with a mixed number: leave the fractions as mixed numbers, find the LCD, change to the same denominator, subtract the numerators and the whole numbers, and reduce to lowest terms.**

Example: Subtract $2\dfrac{1}{8} - \dfrac{3}{6}$

- Find the LCD. For the denominators of 6 and 8, use the LCD of 24.

$$2\frac{1}{8} \text{ becomes } 2\frac{3}{24}$$

$$\frac{3}{6} \text{ becomes } \frac{12}{24}$$

- First, subtract the numerators. Then subtract the whole numbers.

Note: To subtract the larger number (12) from the smaller number (3), you need to borrow 1 or 24/24 from the whole number 2. Then add 24 + 3 = 27, a new numerator. You can now subtract the smaller number (12) from the larger number (27).

$$2\frac{3}{24} = 1\frac{27}{24}$$

$$-\frac{12}{24} = -\frac{12}{24}$$

$$\overline{\qquad\qquad} \quad 1\frac{15}{24} = 1\frac{5}{8}$$

Answer: $1\dfrac{5}{8}$

PRACTICE PROBLEMS

Add and reduce.

1. $\dfrac{5}{11} + \dfrac{9}{11} + \dfrac{13}{11} = $ _____

2. $\dfrac{7}{16} + \dfrac{3}{8} = $ _____

3. $\dfrac{4}{6} + 3\dfrac{1}{8} = $ _____

4. $\dfrac{11}{15} + \dfrac{14}{45} = $ _____

5. $\dfrac{5}{20} + \dfrac{8}{20} + \dfrac{13}{20} = $ _____

6. $\dfrac{9}{19} + 1 = $ _____

7. $\dfrac{4}{7} + \dfrac{9}{14} = $ _____

8. $10 + \dfrac{1}{9} + \dfrac{2}{5} = $ _____

9. $\dfrac{17}{24} + \dfrac{11}{12} = $ _____

10. $\dfrac{4}{5} + \dfrac{1}{10} + \dfrac{2}{3} = $ _____

Subtract and reduce.

11. $\dfrac{6}{7} - \dfrac{3}{7} = $ _____

12. $\dfrac{8}{9} - \dfrac{4}{9} =$ _____

13. $\dfrac{3}{5} - \dfrac{1}{6} =$ _____

14. $\dfrac{3}{4} - \dfrac{2}{9} =$ _____

15. $6\dfrac{3}{7} - \dfrac{2}{3} =$ _____

16. $2\dfrac{1}{6} - 3\dfrac{1}{4} =$ _____

Multiplication of Fractions

Multiplying a Fraction by Another Fraction

> **RULE:** To multiply fractions: multiply the numerators, multiply the denominators, and reduce the product to lowest terms. Reducing can be done before multiplying to make calculations easier. *Remember:* when multiplying a fraction and a whole number, place a one (1) under the whole number so it is expressed as a fraction.

Examples:

$$\frac{3}{4} \times \frac{2}{3} = \frac{3 \times 2}{4 \times 3} = \frac{6}{12} = \frac{1}{2}$$

$$\frac{1}{2} \times \frac{2}{3} = \frac{1 \times 2}{2 \times 3} = \frac{2}{6} = \frac{1}{3}$$

This method of multiplying fractions is sometimes called the "long form." There is also a "short-cut" method for multiplying fractions, called "cancellation." With cancellation, you actually simplify the numbers *before* you multiply by reducing the numbers to the lowest terms. The value stays the same. Look at the example below:

Example: $\dfrac{1}{4} \times \dfrac{8}{15}$

Cancellation can be used because the denominator of the first fraction (4) and the numerator of the second fraction (8) can both be divided by 4 and the value of the fraction does not change. So, if you work the problem, it looks like this:

$$\frac{1}{4} \times \frac{8}{15} = \frac{1}{\cancel{4}_1} \times \frac{\cancel{8}^{\,2}}{15}$$

Once you have canceled all the numbers and reduced them to the lowest terms, you can then multiply the new numerators and the new denominators to get your answer.

$$\frac{1}{1} \times \frac{2}{15} = \frac{2}{15}$$

Answer: $\dfrac{2}{15}$

Multiplying a Fraction by a Mixed Number

When you multiply a fraction by a mixed number, always change the mixed number to an improper fraction before you work the problem. Remember the following rule.

> **RULE: To multiply a fraction by a mixed number: change the mixed number to an improper fraction *before you work the problem.***

Example: $1\frac{1}{2} \times \frac{1}{2}$

Change: $1\frac{1}{2}$ to $\frac{3}{2}$

Multiply: $\frac{3}{2} \times \frac{1}{2} = \frac{3}{4}$

Answer: $\frac{3}{4}$

Example: $1\frac{1}{2} \times 4\frac{1}{2}$

Change: $1\frac{1}{2}$ to $\frac{3}{2}$

Change: $4\frac{1}{2}$ to $\frac{9}{2}$

Multiply: $\frac{3}{2} \times \frac{9}{2} = \frac{27}{4}$ or $6\frac{3}{4}$

Answer: $6\frac{3}{4}$

Division of Fractions

Dividing a Fraction by Another Fraction

Sometimes it is necessary to divide fractions in order to calculate a drug dosage. In any problem, the first fraction (dividend) is *divided by* the second fraction (divisor). The divisor is always to the right of the division sign. With division of fractions, the divisor (5/9) is *always inverted* (9/5) to change the math calculation to multiplication! The answer is called the *quotient*. To divide fractions, follow this rule.

> **RULE:** To divide fractions by another fraction: write your problem as division, invert the divisor, multiply the fractions, and reduce.

Example: Divide $\dfrac{4}{5} \div \dfrac{5}{9}$

- Write your problem as division and invert the divisor.

$$\frac{4}{5} \text{ (dividend)} \div \frac{5}{9} \text{ (divisor)} = \text{quotient}$$

$$\frac{4}{5} \times \frac{9}{5} \left(\text{inverted } \frac{5}{9} \right)$$

- Multiply and reduce. The problem now looks like this:

$$\frac{4}{5} \times \frac{9}{5} = \frac{36}{25} = 1\frac{11}{25}$$

Answer $= 1\dfrac{11}{25}$

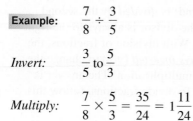

Example: $\dfrac{7}{8} \div \dfrac{3}{5}$

Invert: $\dfrac{3}{5}$ to $\dfrac{5}{3}$

Multiply: $\dfrac{7}{8} \times \dfrac{5}{3} = \dfrac{35}{24} = 1\dfrac{11}{24}$

Answer: $1\dfrac{11}{24}$

Dividing a Fraction by a Mixed Number

> **RULE: To divide fractions that are mixed numbers: change the mixed number to an improper fraction and reduce.**

Example: $\dfrac{3}{6} \div 1\dfrac{2}{5}$

Change: $1\dfrac{2}{5}$ to $\dfrac{7}{5}$

Write: $\dfrac{3}{6} \div \dfrac{7}{5}$

Invert: $\dfrac{7}{5}$ to $\dfrac{5}{7}$

Multiply: $\dfrac{3}{6} \times \dfrac{5}{7} = \dfrac{15}{42}$

Reduce: $\dfrac{15}{42} = \dfrac{5}{14}$

Answer: $\dfrac{5}{14}$

PRACTICE PROBLEMS

Multiplication of Fractions

1. $\dfrac{7}{15} \times \dfrac{8}{12} = $ _____

2. $\dfrac{5}{9} \times \dfrac{3}{7} = $ _____

3. $\dfrac{6}{16} \times \dfrac{2}{5} = $ _____

4. $2\dfrac{7}{10} \times \dfrac{1}{2} = $ _____

5. $3\dfrac{4}{8} \times \dfrac{3}{16} = $ _____

6. $\dfrac{4}{7} \times \dfrac{10}{11} = $ _____

Division of Fractions

7. $\dfrac{3}{4} \div \dfrac{1}{9} = $ _____

8. $\dfrac{6}{13} \div \dfrac{2}{5} = $ _____

9. $\dfrac{8}{12} \div \dfrac{3}{7} = $ _____

10. $12 \div \dfrac{1}{3} = $ _____

11. $8\dfrac{7}{10} \div 15 = $ _____

12. $\dfrac{4}{7} \div \dfrac{2}{13} = $ _____

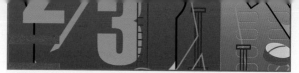

End of Chapter Review

Change the fractions with different denominators to similar fractions by finding the least common denominator:

1. $\dfrac{2}{5}, \dfrac{3}{7}$ _____

2. $\dfrac{7}{5}, \dfrac{4}{20}$ _____

Reduce these fractions to lowest terms:

3. $\dfrac{27}{162} =$ _____

4. $\dfrac{16}{128} =$ _____

Change these improper fractions to mixed numbers:

5. $\dfrac{26}{4} =$ _____

6. $\dfrac{105}{8} =$ _____

Change these mixed numbers to improper fractions:

7. $4\dfrac{6}{11} =$ _____

8. $9\dfrac{2}{23} =$ _____

Reduce these fractions to their lowest terms:

9. $\dfrac{20}{64} =$ _____

10. $\dfrac{16}{128} =$ _____

11. $\dfrac{7}{63} =$ _____

12. $\dfrac{15}{84} =$ _____

Add the following fractions:

13. $\dfrac{1}{9} + \dfrac{7}{9} =$ _____

14. $\dfrac{5}{6} + \dfrac{3}{6} =$ _____

15. $\dfrac{1}{9} + \dfrac{3}{4} =$ _____   **16.** $6\dfrac{5}{6} + \dfrac{3}{8} =$ _____

Subtract the following fractions:

17. $\dfrac{5}{12} - \dfrac{3}{12} =$ _____   **18.** $\dfrac{7}{9} - \dfrac{2}{9} =$ _____

19. $\dfrac{3}{4} - \dfrac{1}{6} =$ _____   **20.** $4\dfrac{6}{10} - \dfrac{3}{8} =$ _____

21. $6\dfrac{3}{8} - 4\dfrac{1}{4} =$ _____   **22.** $\dfrac{9}{12} - \dfrac{7}{24} =$ _____

Multiply the following fractions:

23. $\dfrac{6}{8} \times \dfrac{1}{5} =$ _____   **24.** $\dfrac{9}{11} \times \dfrac{1}{3} =$ _____

25. $2\dfrac{1}{10} \times 6\dfrac{6}{9} =$ _____   **26.** $2\dfrac{2}{7} \times 3\dfrac{4}{8} =$ _____

27. $1\dfrac{5}{11} \times \dfrac{3}{8} =$ _____   **28.** $\dfrac{4}{3} \times 7\dfrac{2}{4} =$ _____

Divide the following fractions:

29. $\dfrac{3}{5} \div \dfrac{7}{20} =$ _____   **30.** $\dfrac{8}{9} \div \dfrac{1}{27} =$ _____

31. $6\dfrac{5}{12} \div \dfrac{15}{24} =$ _____   **32.** $7\dfrac{2}{14} \div 80 =$ _____

33. $16 \div \dfrac{32}{160} =$ _____   **34.** $4 \div \dfrac{8}{9} =$ _____

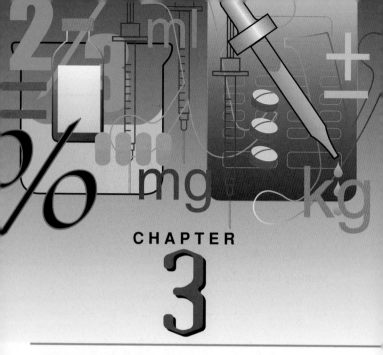

Decimals

LEARNING OBJECTIVES

After completing this chapter, you should be able to:

- Understand the concept of a decimal and decimal fraction.
- Read, write, and compare the value of decimal fractions.
- Add, subtract, multiply, and divide decimals.
- Change fractions to decimals and decimals to fractions.

Medication dosages and other health care measurements are usually prescribed in the metric measure, which is based on the decimal system. Therefore, it is critical that you understand how to read decimals. A serious medication error can occur if the drug dosage written in a decimal format is misread.

A *decimal fraction* is simply a fraction, written in a different format, with a denominator that is any multiple of 10 (10, 100, and 1,000). The decimal point (.) placement determines the decimal's value. See the following examples:

Examples:

Fraction	Decimal	Position to the Right of Decimal	Decimal Point Value
2/10	0.2	1 place	Tenths
3/100	0.03	2 places	Hundredths
4/1,000	0.004	3 places	Thousandths

It is important to remember that numbers to the right of the decimal point are decimal fractions that have a value *less than 1*. Numbers to the left of the decimal point are whole numbers that have a value equal to or *greater than 1*. If there is no whole number before the decimal point, always add a zero (0) to the left of the decimal point to avoid errors when reading the decimal's value. Reading decimals is easy once you understand the concept of decimal values relative to the placement of the decimal point, whole numbers, and decimal fractions. Refer to Figure 3.1 and the following rule.

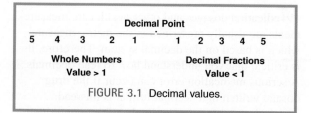

FIGURE 3.1 Decimal values.

RULE: Numbers to the right of the decimal point have a *value less than 1*, and numbers to the left of the decimal point have a *value equal to or greater than 1*.

RULE: To read decimal fractions: read the whole number(s) to the left of the decimal point first, read the decimal point as "and" or "point," and then read the decimal fraction to the right of the decimal point. The zero (0) to the left of the decimal point is not read aloud.

Examples: 0.2 is read as 2 tenths because the number 2 is one position to the right of the decimal point.

0.03 is read as 3 hundredths because the number 3 is two positions to the right of the decimal point.

0.004 is read as 4 thousandths because the number 4 is three positions to the right of the decimal point.

0.150 is read as 15 hundredths because the zero after the 15 does not enhance its value.

Examples:

Read: 5.2   6.03   0.004

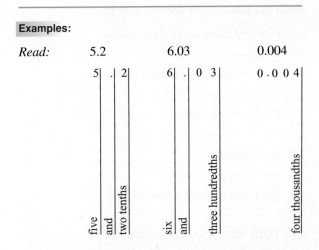

RULE: To write decimal fractions: write the whole number (write zero [0] before the decimal point if there is no whole number), write the decimal point, and then write the decimal fraction. Note: zeros written at the end of the decimal fraction *do not change* the decimal's value.

PRACTICE PROBLEMS

Write the following decimals as you would read them:

1. 10.001 _____

2. 3.0007 _____

3. 0.083 _____

4. 0.153 _____

5. 36.0067 _____   6. 0.0125 _____

7. 125.025 _____   8. 20.075 _____

Write the following in decimal format:

9. Five and thirty-seven thousandths

_____

10. Sixty-four and seven hundredths

_____

11. Twenty thousandths

_____

12. Four tenths

_____

13. Eight and sixty-four thousandths

_____

14. Thirty-three and seven tenths

_____

15. Fifteen thousandths

_____

16. One tenth

_____

Comparing Decimal Values

Understanding which decimals are larger or smaller helps prevent serious medication dosage errors. If a patient was prescribed 0.1 mg of a drug, you wouldn't give 0.2 mg.

RULE: To compare decimal values: the decimal with the largest number in the column to the right of the decimal (tenth place) has the greater value. If both are equal, then apply the rule to the next column (hundredth place). This rule also applies to whole numbers.

Examples:

1. 0.75 is greater than 0.60
2. 0.250 is greater than 0.125
3. 1.36 is greater than 1.25
4. 2.75 is greater than 2.50

PRACTICE PROBLEMS

Select the decimal with the largest value.

1.	0.15	0.25	0.75	_____
2.	0.175	0.186	0.921	_____
3.	1.30	1.35	1.75	_____
4.	2.25	2.40	2.80	_____

Addition of Decimals

RULE: To add decimals: place the decimals in a vertical column with the decimal points directly under one another, add zeros to balance the columns, add the decimals in the same manner as whole numbers are added, and place the decimal in the answer under the aligned decimal points.

Example: *Add:* $0.5 + 3.24 + 8$

$$\begin{array}{r} 0.50 \\ 3.24 \\ +8.00 \end{array}$$

- Add the decimals in the same manner as whole numbers are added.

- Place the decimal in the answer directly under aligned decimal points.

$$\begin{array}{r} 0.50 \\ 3.24 \\ +8.00 \\ \hline 11.74 \end{array}$$

Answer: 11.74

Example: *Add:* $3.9 + 4.7$

$$\begin{array}{r} 3.9 \\ +4.7 \\ \hline 8.6 \end{array}$$

Answer: 8.6

Example: *Add:* $6 + 2.8 + 1.6$

$$\begin{array}{r} 6.0 \\ 2.8 \\ +1.6 \\ \hline 10.4 \end{array}$$

Answer: 10.4

Subtraction of Decimals

> RULE: To subtract decimals: place the decimals in a vertical column with the decimal points directly under one another, add zeros to balance the columns, subtract the decimals in the same manner as whole numbers are subtracted, and place the decimal in the answer under the aligned decimal points.

Example: *Subtract:* 4.1 from 6.2

$$
\begin{array}{r}
6.2 \\
-4.1 \\
\end{array}
$$

- Subtract the decimals in the same manner as whole numbers are subtracted. Place the decimal point in the answer directly under the aligned decimal points.

$$
\begin{array}{r}
6.2 \\
-4.1 \\
\hline
2.1 \\
\end{array}
$$

Answer: 2.1

Example: *Subtract:* $1.32 - 16.84$

$$
\begin{array}{r}
16.84 \\
-1.32 \\
\hline
15.52 \\
\end{array}
$$

Answer: 15.52

Example: *Subtract:* 8.00 − 13.60

$$
\begin{array}{r}
13.60 \\
-8.00 \\
\hline
5.60
\end{array}
$$

Answer: 5.60

Example: *Subtract:* 3.0086 − 7.02

$$
\begin{array}{r}
7.0200 \\
-3.0086 \\
\hline
4.0114
\end{array}
$$

Answer: 4.0114

Multiplication of Decimals

Multiplication of Decimal Numbers

Multiplication of decimals is done using the same method as is used for multiplying whole numbers. The major concern is placement of the decimal point in the product.

> **RULE: To multiply decimals: place the decimals in the same position as whole numbers, multiply, and record the product without decimal points. Count off the number of decimal places *to the right* of both numbers being multiplied, and use that number to place the decimal point in the product. Add zeros on the left if necessary.**

Example: *Multiply:* 6.3 by 7.6

$$
\begin{array}{r}
6.3 \\
\times\ 7.6 \\
\end{array}
$$

- Multiply the decimal numbers as you would multiply whole numbers. Write down the product without the decimal point.

$$
\begin{array}{r}
6.3 \\
\times\ 7.6 \\
\hline
378 \\
441 \\
\hline
4{,}788\ \text{(product)}
\end{array}
$$

- Count off the number of decimal places *to the right* of the decimals in the two numbers being multiplied. In this case, there are two places. Count off the total number of places in the product.

6.3	one place to right of decimal
× 7.6	+ one place to right of decimal
378	
441	
47.88	two places, counting right to left

Answer: 47.88

Multiplication by 10, 100, or 1,000

Multiplying by 10, 100, or 1,000 is a fast and easy way to calculate dosage problems. Simply move the

TABLE 3.1   Multiplying by 10, 100, or 1,000

MULTIPLIER	NUMBER OF ZEROS	MOVE THE DECIMAL TO THE RIGHT
10	1	1 place
100	2	2 places
1,000	3	3 places

decimal point the same number of places to the right as there are zeros in the multiplier. See Table 3.1.

Example: 0.712×10. There is one zero in the multiplier of 10. Move the decimal one place to the right for an answer of 7.12.

$$0.712 = 0.712 = 7.12$$

Example: $0.08 \times 1{,}000$. There are three zeros in the multiplier of 1,000. Move the decimal three places to the right for an answer of 80.

$$0.08 = 0.080 = 80$$

Division of Decimals

Division of Decimal Numbers

To divide decimals, use the same method you would use to divide whole numbers.

When you divide decimals, the most important thing to remember is movement and placement of the decimal point in the divisor (number divided by), dividend (number divided), and quotient (product).

$$\text{Divisor } \overline{)\text{Dividend}}^{\text{Quotient}} \qquad \frac{\text{Dividend}}{\text{Divisor}} = \text{Quotient}$$

$$8\overline{)64}^{8} \qquad \frac{64}{8} = 8$$

> ● **RULE: To divide a decimal by a whole number: place the decimal point in the quotient directly above the decimal point in the dividend.**

Example: $25.5 \div 5$

$$5\overline{)25.5}^{5.1 \text{ (quotient)}}$$
$$\underline{25}$$
$$5$$
$$\underline{5}$$

Answer: 5.1

> ● **RULE: To divide a decimal by a decimal: make the decimal number in the divisor a whole number *first*, move the decimal point in the dividend the same number of places that you moved the decimal point in the divisor, place the decimal point in the quotient directly above the decimal point in the dividend, and add a zero in front of the decimal point.**

Example: To divide 0.32 by 1.6, make 1.6 a whole number (16) by moving the decimal point one place to the right. Move the decimal point in the dividend (0.32) the same number of places (one) that you moved the decimal point in the divisor.

Divide: 3.2 by 16

$$
\begin{array}{r}
.2 \\
16\overline{)3{\uparrow}2} \\
\underline{3.2}
\end{array}
$$

Answer: 0.2

Division by 10, 100, or 1,000

Dividing by 10, 100, or 1,000 is fast and easy. Just move the decimal point the same number of places *to the left* as there are zeros in the divisor. See Table 3.2.

Example: $0.09 \div 10$. Move the decimal one place to the left for an answer of 0.009.

$$0.09 = .009 = 0.009$$
$$\underset{\text{L\_J}}{}$$

TABLE 3.2 Dividing by 10, 100, or 1,000

DIVISOR	NUMBER OF ZEROS	MOVE THE DECIMAL TO THE LEFT
10	1	1 place
100	2	2 places
1,000	3	3 places

PRACTICE PROBLEMS

Add the following decimals:

1. $16.4 + 21.8 = $ _____

2. $0.009 + 18.4 = $ _____

3. $67.541 + 17.1 = $ _____

4. $0.27 + 1.64 = $ _____

5. $1.01 + 18.9 = $ _____

6. $26.07 + 0.0795 = $ _____

Subtract the following decimals:

7. $366.18 - 122.6 = $ _____

8. $107.16 - 56.1 = $ _____

9. $16.19 - 3.86 = $ _____

10. $15.79 - 9.11 = $ _____

11. $148.22 - 81.97 = $ _____

12. $2.46 - 1.34 = $ _____

Multiply the following decimals:

13. $1.86 \times 12.1 = $ _____

14. $0.89 \times 7.65 = $ _____

15. $13 \times 7.8 = $ _____

16. $10.65 \times 100 = $ _____

17. $19.4 \times 2.16 = $ _____

18. $5.33 \times 1.49 = $ _____

19. $16 \times 9.002 =$ _____

20. $54 \times 7.41 =$ _____

Divide the following decimals:

21. $63.8 \div 0.09 =$ _____

22. $39.7 \div 1.3 =$ _____

23. $98.4 \div 1,000 =$ _____

24. $0.008 \div 10 =$ _____

25. $41 \div 4.4 =$ _____

26. $18.61 \div 7.01 =$ _____

27. $134 \div 12.3 =$ _____

28. $99 \div 7.7 =$ _____

Changing Fractions to Decimals

When changing a fraction to a decimal, the numerator of the fraction (1) is divided by the denominator (5). If a numerator does not divide evenly into the denominator, then work the division to three places.

$$\frac{1}{5} = \frac{\text{numerator}}{\text{denominator}} \quad \begin{array}{c}\text{becomes}\\\text{becomes}\end{array} \quad \frac{\text{dividend}}{\text{divisor}} = \frac{1}{5} = 5\overline{)1}$$

> **RULE:** To convert a fraction to a decimal: rewrite the fraction in division format, place a decimal point after the whole number in the dividend, add zeros, place the decimal point in the quotient directly above the decimal point in the dividend, and divide the number by the denominator. Carry out to three places.

Example: Change $\frac{1}{5}$ to a decimal.

- Place a decimal point in the whole number in the dividend.

- Align decimal point in quotient.

- Divide number by denominator and add zeros, if necessary.

$$\frac{1}{5} = \begin{array}{r} 0.2 \\ 5\overline{)1.0} \end{array}$$

Answer: 0.2

Example: *Convert:* $\dfrac{1}{6} = \begin{array}{r} 0.166 \\ 6\overline{)1.000} \\ \underline{6} \\ 40 \\ \underline{36} \\ 40 \\ \underline{36} \\ 4 \end{array}$

Answer: 0.166

Example:

Convert: $\dfrac{1}{8} = 1 \div 8 = 8\overline{)1}$ $\begin{array}{r} .125 \\ 8\overline{)1.000} \\ \underline{8} \\ 20 \\ \underline{16} \\ 40 \\ \underline{40} \end{array}$

Answer: 0.125

Example:

Convert: $\dfrac{5}{20} = \dfrac{1}{4} = 1 \div 4 = 4\overline{)1}$

$$\begin{array}{r} .25 \\ 4\overline{)1.00} \\ \underline{8} \\ 20 \\ \underline{20} \end{array}$$

Answer: 0.25

Example:

Convert: $\dfrac{6}{30} = \dfrac{1}{5} = 1 \div 5 = 5\overline{)1}$

$$\begin{array}{r} .2 \\ 5\overline{)1.0} \\ \underline{10} \end{array}$$

Answer: 0.2

Changing Decimals to Fractions

RULE: To change a decimal to a fraction: simply read the decimal and then write it as it sounds. Reduce if necessary.

Example: Change 0.75 to a fraction.

Read 0.75 as 75 hundredths

Write as $\dfrac{75}{100}$

Reduce $\dfrac{75}{100}$ to $\dfrac{3}{4}$

Example: Change 0.5 to a fraction.

Read 0.5 as 5 tenths

Write as $\dfrac{5}{10}$

Reduce $\dfrac{5}{10}$ to $\dfrac{1}{2}$

Rounding Off Decimals

Most decimals are "rounded off" to the hundredth place to ensure accuracy of calculations. Because this process is done infrequently in the clinical setting, it is explained in *Appendix B* for those of you who wish to review the steps.

PRACTICE PROBLEMS

Convert the following fractions to decimals:

1. $\dfrac{6}{30}$ _____

2. $\dfrac{8}{64}$ _____

3. $\dfrac{15}{60}$ _____

4. $\dfrac{12}{180}$ _____

5. $\dfrac{16}{240}$ _____

6. $\dfrac{3}{57}$ _____

Convert the following decimals to fractions:

7. 0.007 _____

8. 0.93 _____

9. 0.412 _____

10. 5.03 _____

11. 12.2 _____

12. 0.125 _____

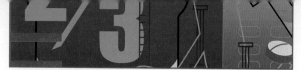

End of Chapter Review

Write the following decimals as you would read them:

1. 5.04 _____
2. 10.65 _____
3. 0.008 _____
4. 18.9 _____

Write the following decimals:

5. Six and eight hundredths

   _____

6. One hundred twenty-four and three tenths

   _____

7. Sixteen and one thousandths

   _____

Solve the following decimal problems:

8. $16.35 + 8.1 =$ _____
9. $0.062 + 59.2 =$ _____
10. $7.006 - 4.23 =$ _____
11. $15.610 - 10.4 =$ _____
12. $27.05 \times 8.3 =$ _____
13. $0.009 \times 14.2 =$ _____
14. $18.75 \div 12 =$ _____
15. $1.070 \div 0.20 =$ _____
16. $12.4 + 3.8 =$ _____
17. $0.893 + 5.88 =$ _____

18. $4.38 - 0.12$ _____

19. $12.78 - 4.31$ _____

20. 38.02×89.1 _____

21. 12.9×0.06 _____

22. $23.56 \div 0.024$ _____

23. $2.109 \div 6.43$ _____

Convert the following fractions to decimals and decimals to fractions:

24. $\dfrac{6}{10}$ _____   30. $\dfrac{8}{20}$ _____

25. $\dfrac{12}{84}$ _____   31. $\dfrac{2}{9}$ _____

26. $\dfrac{3}{4}$ _____   32. $\dfrac{4}{5}$ _____

27. 0.45 _____   33. 6.8 _____

28. 0.75 _____   34. 1.35 _____

29. 0.06 _____   35. 8.5 _____

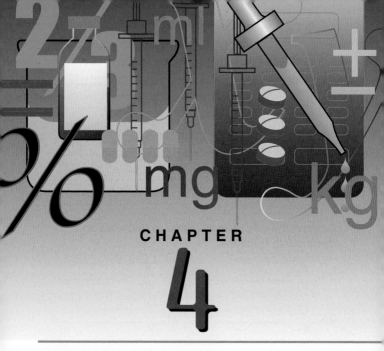

Percent, Ratio, and Proportion

LEARNING OBJECTIVES

After completing this chapter, you should be able to:

- Define the term *percent*.
- Change a percent to a fraction and a fraction to a percent.
- Change a percent to a decimal and a decimal to a percent.
- Determine what percentage one number is of another number.

LEARNING OBJECTIVES (continued)

- Define the terms *ratio* and *proportion*.
- Solve for *x* using ratio and proportion in both the fraction and colon format.

The use of percentages is common in the medical and nursing professions. Physicians prescribe solutions for external application (soaks, compresses) as well as internal use (gargling, irrigations, intravenous infusions). Nurses find themselves, sometimes daily, working with drugs and solutions prepared in percentage strength. It is important to understand that a percent means parts per one hundred (100).

Percents

A *percent*:

- Refers to a number of parts of something, relative to the whole or 100 parts.
- Is a fraction. The denominator is 100; the numerator is the number before the % symbol.
- Is written with the symbol %, which means 100.

Example: $5\% = \dfrac{5}{100} = \dfrac{5 \text{ parts}}{100 \text{ parts}}$

Percents are commonly used when intravenous solutions are prescribed; e.g., 0.25% and 0.45%. These % solutions refer to the grams of the solute or

solid, per 100 parts of solution.
Percents can be written as:

A fraction with a denominator of 100
(1/4%).

A decimal, by taking the unit to the
hundredth part (0.25%).

The *percent symbol* can be found with:

- A whole number   20%
- A fraction number   1/2%
- A mixed number   20 1/2%
- A decimal number   20.5%

Fractions and Percents

Sometimes it is necessary to change a percent to a
fraction or a fraction to a percent to make dosage
calculations easier.

Changing a Percent to a Fraction

> **RULE:** To change a percent to a fraction: drop the % symbol,
> divide the number (new numerator) by 100 (denominator),
> reduce, and change to a mixed number, if necessary.

Example: Change 20% to a fraction

- Drop the % symbol: 20% now becomes
  20.

- This number (20) now becomes the
  fraction's new numerator.

- Place this new numerator (20) over 100 (the denominator will always be 100).

- Reduce the fraction to lowest terms.

- Change to a mixed number if necessary.

Example: *Change: 40%*

$$40\% = 40 = \frac{40}{100}$$

Reduce: $\dfrac{40}{100} = \dfrac{2}{5}$

Answer: $\dfrac{2}{5}$

Example: *Change: $1\dfrac{1}{2}\%$*

$$1\frac{1}{2}\% = 1\frac{1}{2} = \frac{1\frac{1}{2}}{100} = \frac{\frac{3}{2}}{100}$$

$$\frac{3}{2} \div 100 = \frac{3}{2} \times \frac{1}{100} = \frac{3}{200} = 66\frac{2}{3}$$

Answer: $66\dfrac{2}{3}$

Changing a Fraction to a Percent

RULE: To change a fraction to a percent: multiply the fraction by 100 (change any mixed number to an improper fraction *before multiplying by 100*), reduce, and add the % symbol.

Example: *Change:* $\frac{1}{2} = ?$

$$\frac{1}{2} \times \frac{100}{1} = \frac{100}{2} = \frac{50}{1}$$

$$\frac{50}{1} = 50$$

Add % symbol: 50%

Answer: 50%

Example: *Change:* $\frac{3}{4} = ?$

$$\frac{3}{\cancel{4}_1} \times \cancel{100}^{25} = \frac{75}{1} = 75$$

Add % symbol: 75%

Answer: 75%

Example: *Change:* $\frac{3}{5} = ?$

$$\frac{3}{5} \times 100 = \frac{3}{\cancel{5}_1} \times \cancel{100}^{20}_1 = 60$$

Add % symbol: 60%

Answer: 60%

Example: *Change:* $6\frac{1}{2} = ?$

$$6\frac{1}{2} \times 100$$

Change $6\frac{1}{2}$ to an improper fraction.

$$6\frac{1}{2} = \frac{13}{2}$$

$$\frac{13}{2} \times 100 = \frac{13}{2_1} \times \overset{50}{100} = 650$$

Add % symbol: 650%

Answer: 650%

PRACTICE PROBLEMS

Change the following percents to fractions:

1. 15% _____
2. 30% _____
3. 50% _____
4. 75% _____
5. 25% _____
6. 60% _____

Change the following fractions to percents:

7. $\frac{1}{3}$ _____
8. $\frac{2}{3}$ _____
9. $\frac{1}{5}$ _____
10. $\frac{3}{4}$ _____
11. $\frac{2}{5}$ _____
12. $\frac{1}{4}$ _____

Decimals and Percents

Sometimes it is necessary to change a percent to a decimal or a decimal to a percent to make dosage calculations easier.

Changing a Percent to a Decimal

> **RULE:** To change a percent to a decimal: drop the % symbol (when you drop the % symbol from the whole number, a decimal point takes the place of the symbol), divide the remaining number by 100 by moving the decimal point *two places to the left,* and add zeros if necessary.

Example: *Change:* 68%   Drop the % symbol.

68.0 = .68. = 0.68   Move the decimal.
                             Add a zero.

Answer: 0.68

Example: *Change:* 36%

36% = 36% = 36.   Decimal replaces
                  ↑   % symbol.

36. = .36. = 0.36   Move the decimal.
                             Add a zero.

Answer: 0.36

Example: *Change:* 14.1%   Drop the %
                                        symbol.

              14.1% = 14.1% = 14.1   Move the
                                        decimal.

              14.1 = .14.1 = 0.141   Add a zero.
                     └─┘

                                        Answer: 0.141

Changing a Decimal to a Percent

> **RULE:** To change a decimal to a percent: multiply the decimal by 100 by moving the decimal point two places to the right, and add the % symbol and zeros if needed.

Example: *Change:* 3.19

              3.19 = 3.19. = 319   Move the decimal.
                     └──↑

              Add the % symbol.

                                        Answer: 319%

Example: *Change:* 1.61

              1.61 × 100 = 1.61. = 161   Move the
                           └──↑   decimal.

              Add the % symbol.

                                        Answer: 161%

Example: *Change:* 0.5

$0.5 \times 100 = 0.50 = 50$

Add the % symbol.

Note: To move the decimal point two places to the right, you need to add a zero.

Answer: 50%

Percentage One Number Is of Another Number

> **RULE: To determine what percentage one number is of another number: make a fraction using the number following "what percent of" as the denominator, use the remaining number as the numerator, change the fraction to a decimal, and then change the decimal to a percent.**

Example: What percent of 40 is 10?

Convert to a fraction: $\dfrac{10}{40}$

Change to a decimal: $\dfrac{10}{40} = \dfrac{1}{4} = 0.25$

Change to a percent: $0.25 = 25\%$

Example: What percent of 60 is 20?

Convert to a fraction: $\dfrac{20}{60}$

*Change to
a decimal:* $\dfrac{20}{60} = \dfrac{2}{6} = \dfrac{1}{3} = 0.33$

*Change to
a percent:* $0.33 = 33\%$

PRACTICE PROBLEMS

Change the following percents to decimals:

1. 15% _____   2. 25% _____

3. 59% _____   4. 80% _____

Change the following decimals to percents:

5. 0.25 _____   6. 0.45 _____

7. 0.60 _____   8. 0.85 _____

Determine the percentage one number is of
another number.

9. What percent of 90 is 15? _____

10. What percent of 4 is 1/2? _____

11. What percent of 25 is 5? _____

12. What percent of 180 is 60? _____

Ratio and Proportion

A ratio is the same as a fraction: it indicates division. A
ratio is used to express a relationship between one unit
or part of the whole. A slash (/) or colon (:) is used to
indicate division, and both are read as "is to" or "per."

The *numerator (N) of the fraction is always to the left* of the colon or slash, and the *denominator (D) of the fraction is always to the right* of the colon or slash.

With medications, a ratio usually refers to the weight of a drug (e.g., grams) in a solution (e.g., mL). Therefore, 50 mg/mL = 50 mg of a drug (solute) in 1 mL of a liquid (solution). For the ratio of 1 part to a total of 2 parts, you can write 1:2 or 1/2.

Examples: $1:2 = 1/2 = \dfrac{1}{2}$

$2:5 = 2/5 = \dfrac{2}{5}$

$3:6 = 3/6 = \dfrac{3}{6} = \dfrac{1}{2}$

A Proportion Expressed as a Fraction

A *proportion* is two ratios that are equal. A proportion can be written in the fraction or colon format. In the *fraction format*, the numerator and the denominator of one fraction have the same relationship as the numerator and denominator of another fraction (they are equivalent). The equals symbol (=) is read as "as" or "equals."

Example: $\left.\dfrac{1}{3} = \dfrac{3}{9}\right\}$ 1 is to 3 as 3 is to 9

A Proportion Expressed in the Colon Format

In the *colon format*, the ratio to the left of the double colon is equal to the ratio to the right of the double colon. The double colon (::) is read as "as." You can also use an equals symbol (=). The first and fourth terms are called *extremes* and the second and third terms are called the *means*.

EXTREMES

$$\overbrace{1{:}3 :: 3{:}9}$$

MEANS

Example: 1:3 :: 3:9}   1 is to 3 as 3 is to 9

1:3 = 3:9}   1 is to 3 equals 3 is to 9

RULE: To verify that two ratios are equal: multiply the means and then multiply the extremes. The product of the means must always equal the product of the extremes.

Example: 1:3 :: 3:9

$$\underbrace{1{:}3 :: 3{:}9}$$

$1 \times 9 = 9$

$3 \times 3 = 9$

$9 = 9$

Answer: 9

> **RULE:** To verify that two fractions are equal: cross-multiply the numerator of each fraction by its opposite denominator and the products will be equal.

Example: $\dfrac{1}{3} : \dfrac{3}{9}$

$$\dfrac{1}{3} \diagdown\diagup \dfrac{3}{9}$$

$$1 \times 9 = 9$$

$$3 \times 3 = 9$$

$$9 = 9$$

Answer: 9

Use of Ratio and Proportion: Solving for *x*

To review, a *ratio* expresses the relationship of one unit/quantity to another. A *proportion* expresses the relationship between two ratios that are equal. Sometimes you will have to solve a proportion problem with one unknown quantity, known as *x*. If the proportion is written in the colon format, multiply the means and then the extremes. Try to keep the unknown *x* on the left. If the proportion is written in the fraction format, you need to cross-multiply and then divide to solve for *x*.

Solving for x Using a Fraction Format

> **RULE: To solve for *x*:** cross-multiply the numerator of each fraction by its opposite denominator, remembering to *keep the x on the left*. Divide both sides of the equation by the number before the *x*.

Examples:

$$\frac{2}{5} = \frac{x}{20} \qquad 5x = 40 \qquad x = 8$$

$$\frac{1/2}{10} = \frac{x}{40} \qquad 10x = 20 \qquad x = 2$$

$$\frac{36}{12} = \frac{x}{2} \qquad 12x = 72 \qquad x = 6$$

Example:

$$\frac{1}{3} = \frac{x}{9} \qquad x = \text{unknown}$$

Cross-multiply:

$$3 \times x = 9 \times 1$$

$$3x = 9$$

Divide both sides of the equation by the number before the *x* (3).

Divide:

$$\frac{^1\cancel{3}x}{\cancel{3}_1} = \frac{\cancel{9}^3}{\cancel{3}_1}$$

Reduce:

$$x = \frac{3}{1}$$

$$x = 3$$

Answer: 3

Note: Because the number *before* the x is the same in the numerator and denominator of one ratio, these numbers will cross themselves out and equal 1. Therefore, a shortcut is to *move the number before the x* to the denominator *on the opposite side.* This quick process is especially important when solving for x in dosage calculation problems.

Solving for x Using a Colon Format

> **RULE: To solve for x:** write what you have or know in the colon format (25 : 5), and then write what you desire or the unknown in colon format (50 : x). Therefore, 25 : 5 = 50 : x. Multiply the extremes (25 × x), which keeps the x on the left, and then multiply the means (5 × 50). Then solve for x.

A medication example will be presented next in order to illustrate how to apply the concept of *solving for x*, using ratio and proportion, for drug dosage problems.

Applying the Concept of Solving for x Using a Sample Dosage Problem

Frequently in dosage calculation problems, one quantity is known (100 mg/mL), and it is necessary to find an unknown quantity because the physician has ordered something different from what is available (75 mg). The unknown quantity (? mL necessary to give 75 mg) is identified as x.

The following medication problem will be solved using both the fraction and decimal/colon format.

Example: Demerol, 75 mg, is prescribed for post-operative pain. The medication is available as 100 mg/mL. To administer the prescribed dose of 75 mg, the nurse would give _____ mL.

- For the fraction format, always write down what is available or *what you have.* You are expressing the ratio relationship of one quantity (mg) to another quantity (mL). *Remember,* the unit of measurement in the numerator of the fraction must be the same for both fractions. The unit of measurement in the denominator of the fraction also must be the same for both fractions.

$$\frac{100 \text{ mg}}{1 \text{ mL}}$$

- Complete the proportion by writing down what you desire (what the physician had ordered), making sure that the numerators are like units and the denominators are like units in the fraction ratios used.

$$\frac{\text{mg}}{\text{mL}} :: \frac{\text{mg}}{\text{mL}} = \frac{100 \text{ mg}}{1 \text{ mL}} :: \frac{75 \text{ mg}}{x \text{ mL}}$$

- Cross-multiply the numerator of each fraction by its opposite denominator and *drop the terms used for units of measurement.*

$$\frac{100 \text{ mg}}{1 \text{ mL}} \diagdown \diagup \frac{75 \text{ mg}}{x \text{ mL}}$$

- Complete the proportion:

$$100 \times x = 75 \times 1$$
$$100x = 75$$

- Solve for x by dividing both sides of the equation by the number before x. In this case, the number before x is 100, so divide both sides of the equation by 100. Convert your answer to a decimal, which is easier to work with than a fraction. Refer to pages 71–72 to review the traditional and abbreviated methods for solving for x. For the purpose of brevity, an abbreviated method will be used throughout the remainder of the book.

$$\frac{100x}{100} = \frac{75}{100}$$

$$x = \frac{75}{100}$$

- Reduce: $x = \dfrac{3}{4}$ mL or 0.75 mL

Answer: 3/4 or 0.75 mL

Example: Demerol in 75 mg is prescribed for postoperative pain. The medication is available as 100 mg/mL. To administer the prescribed dose of 75 mg, the nurse would have to give _____ mL.

- For the decimal/colon format, always write down what is available or *what you have. Remember,* the unit of measurement to the left of the colon must be the same for both ratios; the unit of measurement to the right of the colon must be the same for both ratios. For this example, you should write:

$$100 \text{ mg} : 1 \text{ mL}$$

• Complete the proportion by writing down *what you desire*, making sure that both ratios are written in the same format.

$$100 \text{ mg} : 1 \text{ mL} = 75 \text{ mg} : x \text{ mL}$$

• Multiply the extremes:

$$\overline{\quad\quad \text{EXTREMES} \quad\quad}$$
$$100 \text{ mg} : 1 \text{ mL} :: 75 \text{ mg} : x \text{ mL}$$

$$(100 \text{ mg} \times x \text{ mL} = \quad\quad)$$

• Multiply the means:

$$100 \text{ mg} : 1 \text{ mL} :: 75 \text{ mg} : x \text{ mL}$$
$$\underline{\quad \text{MEANS} \quad}$$

$$(\quad\quad\quad = 75 \text{ mg} \times 1 \text{ mL})$$

• Complete the equation (100 mg × *x* mL = 75 mg × 1 mL) and *drop the units of measurement*.

$$100x = 75$$

• Solve for *x*. (Remember: divide both sides of the equation by the number before *x* [100].) Convert your answer to a decimal.

$$\frac{100x}{100} = \frac{75}{100}$$

$$\frac{\cancel{100}x}{\cancel{100}} = \frac{75}{100}$$

- Reduce: $x = \dfrac{3}{4}$ mL or 0.75 mL

Answer: 3/4 or 0.75 mL

Verifying Accuracy

> **RULE:** To verify the accuracy of an answer obtained by solving for *x*, determine that the sum products are equal.

Verify the accuracy of the answer, $x = 0.75$ mL.

- For the *fraction format,* multiply the numerator of each ratio by its opposite denominator. The sum products will be equal.

$$\frac{100 \text{ mg}}{1 \text{ mL}} :: \frac{75 \text{ mg}}{\dfrac{3}{4} \text{ mL}}$$

$$\left.\begin{array}{l} ^{25}\cancel{100} \times \dfrac{3}{\cancel{4}_1} = 75 \\[2mm] 1 \times 75 = 75 \end{array}\right\} \begin{array}{l} \text{Sum products} \\ \text{are equal} \end{array}$$

- For the *colon format,* multiply the extremes and then multiply the means. The product of the means will equal the product of the extremes.

$$\overbrace{100 \text{ mg} : 1 \text{ mL} :: 75 \text{ mg} : x \text{ mL}}^{\text{EXTREMES}}$$

MEANS

$$75 \times 1 \text{ mL} = 75$$

$$\left. 100 \times \frac{3}{4} = \frac{\cancel{100}^{25}}{1} \times \frac{3}{\cancel{4}_1} = 75 \right\} \begin{array}{l} \text{Sum products} \\ \text{are equal} \end{array}$$

Critical Thinking Check:

If 75 mg is prescribed and 100 mg/mL is available, does it seem logical that the quantity to be given would be less than 1.0 mL? _____ **Yes or No?**

PRACTICE PROBLEMS

Write the following relationships in ratio form, using both the fraction and colon format:

1. Pediatric drops contain 50 mg/5 mL.

2. There are 325 mg in each tablet.

3. A liter of IV solution contains 2 ampules of multivitamins.

4. A capsule contains 250 mg of a drug.

Write the following relationships as proportions, using both the fraction and colon format:

5. Each tablet contains 5 grains of a drug. The nurse is to give 3 tablets equal to 15 grains.

6. A drug is available in 0.2-mg tablets. A patient is prescribed 0.4 mg/day provided by 2 tablets.

7. A syrup contains 10 mg/5 mL. A patient is to take 30 mg or 15 mL during a 24-hour period.

Use ratio and proportion to solve for *x*.

8. $\dfrac{4}{12} = \dfrac{3}{x}$ _____

9. $\dfrac{6}{x} = \dfrac{9}{27}$ _____

10. $\dfrac{2}{7} = \dfrac{x}{14}$ _____

11. $\dfrac{5}{25} = \dfrac{10}{x}$ _____

12. If 50 mg of a drug is available in 1 mL of solution, how many milliliters would contain 40 mg?

    Set up ratio: proportion and solve for *x:* _____

13. A drug is available as 25 mg/mL.

    To give 1.5 mL, you would give _____ mg.

    Set up ratio: proportion and solve for *x:* _____

14. A tablet contains 0.125 mg.

    The nurse gave 2 tablets or _____ mg.

    Set up ratio: proportion and solve for *x:* _____

15. An oral liquid is available as 1 gram in each 5 mL.

    The nurse gave 15 mL or _____ grams.

    Set up ratio: proportion and solve for *x:* _____

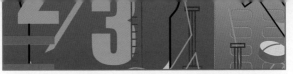

End of Unit 1 Review

Change the following:

Percent	Fraction	Decimal
1. _____	1/6	_____
2. _____	_____	0.25
3. 6.4%	_____	_____
4. 21%	_____	_____
5. _____	2/5	_____
6. _____	_____	1.62
7. _____	_____	0.27
8. 5 1/4%	_____	_____
9. _____	9/2	_____
10. 8 3/9%	_____	_____
11. 1%	_____	_____
12. _____	6/7	_____
13. _____	18/4	_____
14. _____	_____	1.5
15. _____	_____	0.72

Write the following ratios in fraction and colon format:

16. A tablet contains 10 mg of a drug.

_____ fraction _____ colon

17. A liquid is available for injection as 10 units in each milliliter.

   _____ fraction _____ colon

18. A physician ordered 200 mg of a drug per kilogram of body weight.

   _____ fraction _____ colon

19. The physician ordered 300 mg of a drug, which was available in 100-mg tablets.

   _____ fraction _____ colon

20. A physician ordered 500 mg of a drug. The medication was available in 250-mg tablets.

   _____ fraction _____ colon

21. A drug is available in 0.075-mg tablets. A physician ordered 0.15 mg daily.

   _____ fraction _____ colon

22. A physician ordered 500 mg of a liquid medication that was available as 250 mg/0.5 mL.

   _____ fraction _____ colon

Solve for *x*, using ratios and proportions.

23. If $\dfrac{1}{50} = \dfrac{x}{40}$ then $x =$

24. If $\dfrac{6}{18} = \dfrac{2}{x}$ then $x =$

25. If $\dfrac{x}{12} = \dfrac{9}{24}$ then $x =$

26. If $\dfrac{3}{9} = \dfrac{x}{18}$ then $x =$

Solve for x for the remaining problems and verify your answers using a fraction or colon format: use a *critical thinking check* to evaluate the logic of your answer.

27. The physician prescribed 10 mg of a day. The medication was available as 20 mg/mL. The nurse would give _____ mL.

    Verify your answer: _____

    Critical Thinking Check:

    If one-half the available dosage is prescribed, then does it seem logical that the quantity to be given would be less than 1.0 mL? _____ **Yes or No?**

28. The physician prescribed 25 mg of a syrup to be given every 3 hours for pain as needed. The syrup was available as 50 mg/5 mL. To give 25 mg, the nurse would give _____ mL.

    Verify your answer: _____

    Critical Thinking Check:

    If one-half the available dosage (50 mg/5 mL) is prescribed, then does it seem logical that the quantity to be given would be less than 3 mL? _____ **Yes or No?**

29. The physician ordered 1.5 mg of an injectable liquid. The medication was available as 3.0 mg/mL. The nurse would give _____ mL.

    Verify your answer: _____

    Critical Thinking Check:

    If one-half the available dosage is prescribed (3 mg/1 mL), then does it seem logical that the quantity to be given would be less than 1 mL? _____
    Yes or No?

30. The physician prescribed 25 mg of a one-dose injectable liquid. The drug was available as 20 mg/2 mL. The nurse would give _____ mL.

    Verify your answer: _____

    Critical Thinking Check:

    If an additional 25% of the available dosage (20 mg/2 mL) is prescribed, does it seem logical that the quantity to be given would be greater than 3 mL? _____ **Yes or No?**

31. The physician prescribed 30 mg of an oral solution available as 20 mg/5 mL. The nurse would give _____ mL.

32. The physician prescribed 40 mg of a solution that was available as 80 mg/15 mL. To give 40 mg, the nurse would give _____ mL.

33. The physician prescribed 7.5 mg of a medication that was available as 15 mg/mL. The nurse would give _____ mL.

34. The physician prescribed 0.6 mg of a medication that was available as 0.4 mg/mL. To give 0.6 mg, the nurse would give _____ mL.

35. The physician prescribed 80 mg of a medication that was available as 100 mg/2 mL. The nurse would give _____ mL.

36. The physician ordered 35 mg of a liquid that was available as 50 mg/mL. The nurse would give _____ mL.

37. The physician ordered 60 mg of a drug that was available as 20 mg/tablet. The nurse would give _____ tablets.

End of Unit 1 Review

Solve the following problems and reduce each answer to its lowest terms.

1. $1/4 + 3/4$ _____
2. $2/3 - 3/5$ _____
3. $1/10 + 3/5$ _____
4. $3/4 - 1/3$ _____
5. $2/6 \times 4/5$ _____
6. $3/8 \times 1/6$ _____
7. $1/50 \times 20/30$ _____
8. $1/100 \times 20/30$ ___
9. $1/3 \div 1/6$ _____
10. $1/10 \div 1/8$ _____
11. $1/12 \div 1/3$ _____
12. $1/15 \div 3/150$ ___

Choose the fraction with the highest value in each of the following.

13. $1/3$ or $1/4$ _____
14. $1/8$ or $1/6$ _____
15. $1/100$ or $1/200$ ___
16. $3/30$ or $5/30$ ___

Solve the following and carry to the nearest hundredths.

17. $1.5 + 1.6$ _____
18. $0.46 + 3.8$ _____
19. $0.6 - 0.2$ _____
20. $6 - 0.32$ _____
21. 0.25×10 _____
22. 0.15×100 ___
23. $7.5 \div 0.45$ _____
24. $8.5 \div 4.5$ _____

Change the following fractions to decimals and
decimals to fractions.

25. 8/10 _____   26. 5/20 _____

27. 3/9 _____   28. 0.5 _____

29. 0.07 _____   30. 1.5 _____

Change the following percents to fractions and
fractions to percents.

31. 25% _____   32. 1/3% _____

33. 0.6% _____   34. 2/5 _____

35. 4 1/2 _____   36. 1/50 _____

Solve for the value of *x* in each ratio and proportion
problem. Reduce all fractions to their lowest terms
or carry all decimals to the hundredths or tenths.
Verify your answers.

37. $3 : x = 4 : 16$ _____

38. $25 : 1.5 = 20 : x$ _____

39. $8 : 1 = 10 : x$ _____

40. $4/5 : 25 = x : 50$ _____

41. $0.25 : 500 = x : 1,000$ _____

42. $x : 20 = 2.5 : 100$ _____

43. $10 : 30 = 60 : x$ _____

44. $1/2 : 8 = 1/8 : x$ _____

45. $3 : x = 9 : 1/3$ _____

46. $125 : 250 = 300 : x$ _____

47. $1/2 : x = 1/4 : 0.8$ _____

48. $1/5 : 10 = 1/10 : x$ _____

49. $1/100 : 5 = 1/150 : x$ _____

50. $15 : x = 25 : 150$ _____

51. $8 : x = 48 : 6$ _____

52. $4 : 8 = x : 0.5$ _____

53. $1.5 : 2 = x : 2.5$ _____

54. $20 : x = 80 : 8$ _____

55. $1/75 : 1/150 = 2 : x$ _____

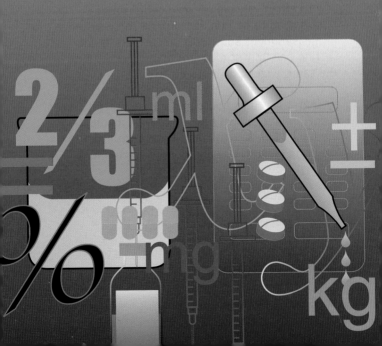

Measurement Systems

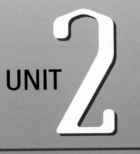

The metric and apothecary systems of weights and measures are in wide use today, as they have been for many years. Although the apothecary system is still used by many health care practitioners, the use of household measurements is becoming more popular, especially with the current shift in health delivery from the institution to the home. These systems have three basic units of measurement: weight, volume, and length. Drugs are commonly prescribed by weight (milligram, gram, grain) and volume (milliliter, ounce). Length is usually used for assessment (inches, millimeters, centimeters).

To effectively deliver medications today, nurses need to be familiar with all three systems of measurement and to become expert at converting one unit of measure to another within the same system, or between two systems. This unit will present the metric and apothecary systems as well as household measurements. The reader will be shown how to convert all measurements. Equivalent values have been listed to facilitate conversions and dosage calculations.

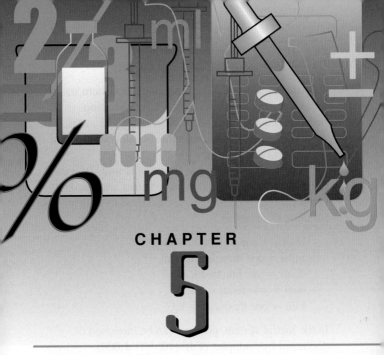

The Metric System

LEARNING OBJECTIVES

After completing this chapter, you should be able to:

- List the common rules for metric notation.
- Distinguish between the three units of measure: length (meter), weight (gram), and volume (liter).
- Make conversions within the metric system.

The metric system is the most popular system used today for drug prescription and administration because it is the most accurate system. The metric system of weights and measures is a decimal system based on multiples of ten.

The metric system has three basic units of measurement: length (meter), volume (liter), and weight (gram). Five common prefixes are used to indicate subunits of measure:

micro = one millionth = mcg*
milli = one thousandth = m
centi = one hundredth = c
deci = one tenth = deci
kilo = one thousand = kg

In the metric system, portions can be increased or decreased by multiples of 10 (10, 100, 1,000). Conversions are achieved by moving the decimal point to the right for multiplication or to the left for division.

1.0 *increased by* 10 = 1.0. = 10

0.1 *decreased by* 10 = 0.1 = 0.01

Common Rules for Metric Notations

⬤ **RULE: Metric abbreviations always follow the unit amount or numbers.**

0.2 mL   10 kg

*Avoid μg for microgram. It is no longer approved by The Joint Commission on the Accreditation of Healthcare Organizations.

> **RULE:** Metric abbreviations are written in lowercase letters except for the word *liter;* the "L" is capitalized.

> g = gram
> mL = milliliter

> **RULE:** Fractional units are expressed as decimal fractions.

> 0.5 mL *not* 1/2 mL

> **RULE:** Zeros are used *in front of* the decimal point, when not preceded by a whole number, to emphasize the decimal. Omit unnecessary zeros so the dosage is not misread.

> 0.5 mL *not* 0.50 mL
> 1 mL *not* 1.0 mL

Meter—Length

A meter is:

- The basic unit of *length*
- Equal to 39.37 inches
- Abbreviated as m

The primary linear measurements used in medicine are centimeters (cm) and millimeters (mm). Centimeters are used for measuring such things as the size of body organs and wounds; millimeters are used for blood

TABLE 5.1 Metric Units of Length

$$1 \text{ meter} = \begin{cases} 10 \text{ decimeters (dm)} \\ 100 \text{ centimeters (cm)} \\ 1{,}000 \text{ millimeters (mm)} \end{cases}$$

1,000 meters = 1 kilometer

pressure measurements. The important units of metric length and abbreviations are found in Table 5.1.

Converting Within the System

Converting or changing units in the metric system is easily done by moving the decimal point. If you choose, you can always use ratio and proportion.

> **RULE:** To move *from a smaller* unit *to a larger* unit within the same system: *divide* by moving the decimal point *to the left* the number of places to be moved (move one place for each increment).

Example: Change millimeters (6,000) to decimeters. To move from milli to deci, you need to move the decimal point two places *to the left*.

60.00. = 60
(milli) = (deci)

Answer: 60 dm

> **RULE:** To move *from a larger* unit *to a smaller* unit within the same system: *multiply* by moving the decimal point *to the right* the number of places to be moved (move one place for each increment of 10).

Example: Change decimeters (80) to centimeters. To move from deci to centi, you need to move the decimal point one place *to the right*.

$$80.0. = 800$$

(deci) = (centi)

Answer: 800 cm

PRACTICE PROBLEMS

Change the following units of metric length:

1. 3.60 cm = _____ m

2. 4.16 m = _____ dm

3. 0.8 mm = _____ cm

4. 2 mm = _____ m

5. 20.5 mm = _____ cm

6. 18 cm = _____ mm

7. 30 dm = _____ mm

8. 2 cm = _____ m

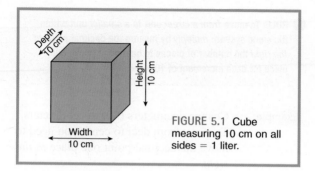

FIGURE 5.1 Cube measuring 10 cm on all sides = 1 liter.

Liter—Volume

A liter is:

- The basic unit of *volume*
- The total volume of liquid in a cube that measures 10 cm × 10 cm × 10 cm (= cm³) (see Figure 5.1)
- Equal to 1,000 mL = 1,000 cubic centimeters (cc)
- Abbreviated as L

The rules for moving from larger to smaller and from smaller to larger units of metric length can also be used for units of metric volume and weight. The units of metric volume can be found in Table 5.2.

TABLE 5.2 Units of Metric Volume

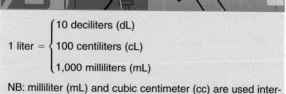

$$1 \text{ liter} = \begin{cases} 10 \text{ deciliters (dL)} \\ 100 \text{ centiliters (cL)} \\ 1,000 \text{ milliliters (mL)} \end{cases}$$

NB: milliliter (mL) and cubic centimeter (cc) are used interchangeably. However, mL should be used (not cc) to avoid medication errors.

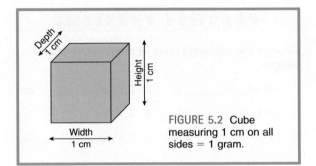

FIGURE 5.2 Cube measuring 1 cm on all sides = 1 gram.

Gram—Weight

A gram is:

- The basic unit of *weight*
- The weight of distilled water in the space of 1 cubic centimeter at a temperature of 4°C
- A cube 1 cm³ (see Figure 5.2)
- Equal to a volume of 1 mL or cc
- Abbreviated as g

The units of metric weight can be found in Table 5.3.

TABLE 5.3 Metric Units of Weight

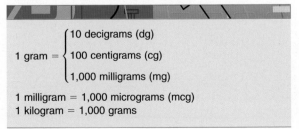

1 gram =	10 decigrams (dg)
	100 centigrams (cg)
	1,000 milligrams (mg)

1 milligram = 1,000 micrograms (mcg)
1 kilogram = 1,000 grams

PRACTICE PROBLEMS

Change the following units of metric volume and weight:

1. 3.6 mL = _____ L   2. 6.17 cL = _____ mL

3. 0.9 L = _____ mL   4. 6.40 cg = _____ mg

5. 1,000 mg = _____ g   6. 0.8 mg = _____ dg

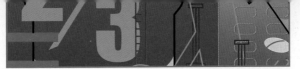

End of Chapter Review

Change the following units of metric length:

1. 7.43 mm = _____ m   2. 0.06 cm = _____ dm

3. 10 km = _____ m   4. 62.17 dm = _____ mm

Change the following units of metric volume:

5. 1.64 mL = _____ dL   6. 0.47 dL = _____ L

7. 10 L = _____ cL   8. 56.9 cL = _____ mL

Change the following units of metric weight:

9. 35.6 mg = _____ g   10. 0.3 g = _____ cg

11. 0.05 g = _____ mg   12. 93 cg = _____ mg

13. 100 mcg = _____ mg   14. 2 mg = _____ mcg

15. 1.0 mcg = _____ mg   16. 7 kg = _____ g

Perform the following miscellaneous conversions:

17. 4 mg = _____ mcg   18. 13 kg = _____ g

19. 2.5 L = _____ mL   20. 0.6 mg = _____ mcg

21. 0.08 g = _____ mg   22. 0.01 mg = _____ mcg

23. 60 mg = _____ g   24. 10.5 mg = _____ mcg

25. 0.5 mL = _____ L   26. 100 mg = _____ dg

27. 3.5 dg = _____ g   28. 3.4 mg = _____ g

29. 30 mg = _____ mcg   30. 13 cg = _____ g

31. 2 kg = _____ g   32. 18 L = _____ mL

33. 450 g = _____ mg   34. 40 mcg = _____ mg

35. 8 L = _____ dL   36. 10 L = _____ cL

37. 46 g = _____ dg   38. 0.5 g = _____ mg

39. 500 mL = _____ L   40. 25 kg = _____ g

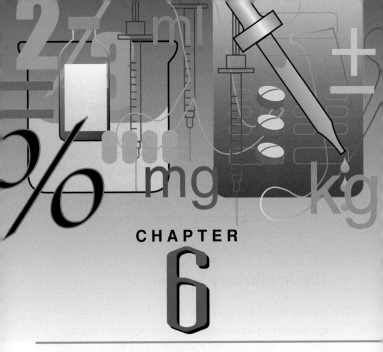

6

The Apothecary System and Household Measurements

LEARNING OBJECTIVES

After completing this chapter, you should be able to:

- List the units of weight and volume for the apothecary system.

107

- List the common quantities of measurement for the household system.
- State the common rules for the apothecary system.
- State the common rules for the household system.
- Identify the symbols used for apothecary measures.
- Identify the symbols used for household measures.
- Use approximate equivalent values and convert between the apothecary system and household measurements.

The Apothecary System

One of the oldest systems of measurement is the apothecary system. Although less popular than the metric system, and not recommended for use, it is still used by physicians, especially for prescribing medications that have been used for many years (e.g., digitalis, aspirin).

The apothecary system uses approximate measures, fractions, Arabic numbers, and Roman numerals (see Appendix A). Three symbols—"gr" for grain, "3" or "dr" for dram, and "3̄" or "oz" for ounce—are common. The symbol for ounce is the same symbol as dram (3), with a "hat" on top (3̄). The small letter "f" refers to fluid.

It is helpful to understand the relationship of a term to the concept of weight and volume. The original standard measurement of a grain was an amount equal to the weight of a grain of wheat. The minim is considered equal to the quantity of water in a drop that also weighs 1 grain. A dram is equal to 4 mL; an ounce is equal to 30 mL.

TABLE 6.1 Apothecary Units of Weight

UNIT	WEIGHT	SYMBOL
Grain*	—	gr
Dram	60 grains	ʒ
Ounce	8 drams	ʒ or oz
Pound	12 ounces†	lb

*The grain is the basic unit.
†A pound in this system is equal to 12 ounces; a pound in the English system is equal to 16 ounces.

TABLE 6.2 Apothecary Units of Volume

UNIT	VOLUME	SYMBOL
Minim*	1 drop of water	m or min
Fluidram†	60 minims	fʒ
Fluidounce†	8 fluidrams	fʒ
Pint	16 fluidounces	pt or O
Quart	2 pints	qt
Gallon	4 quarts	gal or C

*The minim is the basic unit.
†When the substance is known to be a liquid, the term fluid does not have to be used.

The apothecary system has two basic units of measurement: weight and volume (see Tables 6.1 and 6.2).

Common Rules for the Apothecary System

RULE: Lowercase Roman numerals are used to express whole numbers.

$$3 = iii \qquad 6 = vi$$

> **RULE: Arabic numbers are used for larger quantities (except for 5, 20, and 30) or when the amount is written out.**

12   or   twelve drams

> **RULE: The apothecary abbreviation *always goes before* the quantity.**

gr x̄ = 10 grains

ʒ viii = eight drams

> **RULE: Fractional units are used to express quantities that are less than one (gr. 1/3). The symbol ss or s̄s̄ is used for the fraction 1/2.**

Household Measurements

Household measurements are calculated by using containers easily found in the home. Common household measuring devices are those utensils used for cooking, eating, and measuring liquid proportions. They include medicine droppers, teaspoons, tablespoons, cups, and glasses. Because containers in the home differ in design, size, and capacity, it is impossible to establish a standard unit of measure. Patients should always be advised to first use measuring cups or droppers packaged with medications.

TABLE 6.3 Common Household Quantities and Metric Equivalents

UNIT	VOLUME	SYMBOL	METRIC EQUIVALENT
Drop	—	gtt	—
Teaspoon	60 drops	t or tsp	5 mL
Tablespoon	3 teaspoons	T or tbs	15 mL
Ounce	2 tablespoons	oz	30 mL
Tea cup	6 ounces	c	180 mL
Measuring cup	8 ounces	C	240 mL
Pint	16 ounces	pt	500 mL
Quart	2 pints	qt	1,000 mL

The household measurement system is the *least accurate* of all three systems, yet its use will increase as health care continues to move into the home and community. The nurse or health care provider will have to teach the patient/family how to measure the amount of medication prescribed, so every effort needs to be made to be as exact as possible. Refer to Table 6.3.

Probably the *most common* measuring device found in the home is the measuring cup, which calibrates ounces and is available for liquid and dry measures (Figure 6.1). Additionally, many families have a 1-ounce measuring cup that calibrates teaspoons and/or tablespoons (Figure 6.2). Some pharmaceutical companies package 1-ounce measuring cups or calibrated medicine droppers with their over-the-counter medications (NyQuil, Children's Tylenol).

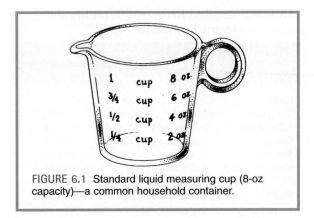

FIGURE 6.1 Standard liquid measuring cup (8-oz capacity)—a common household container.

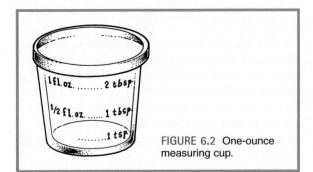

FIGURE 6.2 One-ounce measuring cup.

Common Rules for the Household System

RULE: Arabic whole numbers and fractions *precede* the unit of measure.

¼ cup   8 ounces   3 cups   2 pints

The household system of measurement uses Arabic whole numbers and fractions to precede the unit of measure. Standard cookbook abbreviations are also used (tsp, tbsp, oz). The basic unit of this system is the drop (gtt). A drop is equal to a drop, regardless of the liquid's viscosity (sticky or gummy consistency). Therefore, when medicine needs to be given in drops, a standard dropper should be used. Household measurements are approximate in comparison to the exactness of the metric and apothecary systems. Hospitals use a standard 1-ounce medicine cup (Figure 6.3). These calibrated containers provide metric, apothecary, and household system equivalents.

> **RULE:** When measuring a liquid medication in a household container, determine the container's capacity *prior to preparing* the medication.

When measuring a liquid medication, it is important that the container/dropper be held so the calibrations are at eye level. When a container/dropper is held at eye level, the liquid will appear to be

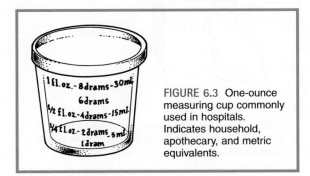

FIGURE 6.3 One-ounce measuring cup commonly used in hospitals. Indicates household, apothecary, and metric equivalents.

uneven or U-shaped. This curve, called a *meniscus,* is caused by surface tension; its shape is influenced by the viscosity of the fluid. When measuring the level of a liquid medication, read the calibration "at the bottom" of the meniscus (Figure 6.4).

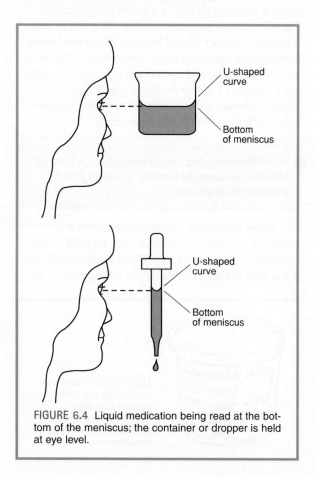

FIGURE 6.4 Liquid medication being read at the bottom of the meniscus; the container or dropper is held at eye level.

Converting Within the Same System

Sometimes it will be necessary to convert or change units *within the same system* for the apothecary system and household measures. These conversions *require the memorization of common equivalents,* which can be found in Tables 6.1, 6.2, and 6.3. There is a standard rule to use to convert units *within the same system,* using ratio and proportion. Converting *between systems* will be covered in the next chapter.

> **RULE: To change units within the same system: determine equivalent values, write down *what you know* followed by *what you desire,* in a fraction or colon format, and solve for *x*.**

Example:

- Select the equivalent values in the system. If you want to know how many ounces there are in 20 drams, look up the equivalent value of 8 drams = 1 ounce (Table 6.1).

- Write down what you know in a colon or fraction format:

$$\frac{8 \text{ drams}}{1 \text{ ounce}} \quad \text{or} \quad 8 \text{ drams} : 1 \text{ ounce}$$

- Write down what you desire in a colon or fraction format to complete the proportion. The numerators and denominators must be the same units of measurement. The unknown unit is referred to as x:

$$\frac{8 \text{ drams}}{1 \text{ ounce}} :: \frac{20 \text{ drams}}{x \text{ ounces}} \quad \text{or}$$

8 drams : 1 ounces :: 20 drams : x ounce

- Cross-multiply (fraction format) or multiply the extremes and then the means (colon format). Drop the terms used for units of measurement.

8 drams $\times$ x ounces = 20 drams $\times$ 1 ounce

$$8x = 20$$

- Solve for x (divide both sides of the equation by the number before the x [8]). You are reducing both sides of the equation.

$$\frac{8x}{8} = \frac{20}{8}$$

$$\frac{8^1 x}{8_1} \quad x = \frac{20^5}{8_2}$$

$$x = \frac{5}{2} = 2\frac{1}{2}$$

Answer: $2\frac{1}{2}$ ounces

Example: Select the equivalent values in the system (see Table 6.3). If you want to know how many ounces there are in 2 tablespoons, look up the equivalent value of 1 ounce = 2 tablespoons.

- Write down *what you know* in a fraction or colon format.

$$\frac{2 \text{ tbs}}{1 \text{ oz}} \quad \text{or} \quad 2 \text{ tbs} : 1 \text{ oz}$$

- Write down *what you desire* in a fraction or colon format to complete the proportion. The unknown unit is referred to as *x*. The numerators and denominators must be the same units of measurement. Consider the fraction format here.

$$\frac{2 \text{ tbs}}{1 \text{ oz}} : \frac{4 \text{ tbs}}{x \text{ oz}} \quad \text{or} \quad 2 \text{ tbs}: 1 \text{ oz} = 4 \text{ tbs}: x \text{ oz}$$

- Cross-multiply or use ratio and proportion to get the following. Drop the terms used for units of measurement.

$$2 \text{ tbs} \times x \text{ oz} = 4 \text{ tbs} \times 1 \text{ oz}$$
$$2x = 4$$

- Solve for *x*:

$$\frac{2x}{2} = \frac{4}{2} \qquad \frac{2^1 x}{2_1} = \frac{4^2}{2_1} \qquad x = 2$$

Answer: 2 ounces

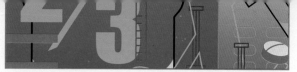

End of Chapter Review

Write the following, using Roman numerals and symbols:

1. 3 grains _____   2. 5 drams _____

3. 8 fluidrams _____   4. 10 minims _____

5. 20 1/2 minims _____   6. 5 pints _____

Solve the following:

7. 8 quarts = _____ gallon(s)

8. f℥ ii = _____ minim(s)

9. f℥ iv = _____ fluidram(s)

10. gr xxx = _____ dram(s)

11. f℥ viii = _____ ounce(s)

12. 4 pints = _____ quart(s)

13. 4 ounces = _____ pint(s)

14. gr xv = _____ dram(s)

15. 1/4 ℥ = _____ dram(s)

16. ℥ s̄s̄ = _____ dram(s)

Convert the following units to their equivalent value:

17. 12 ounces = _____ cup(s)

18. 3 glasses = _____ ounces

19. 6 tablespoons = _____ ounce(s)

20. 2 teaspoons = _____ drops

21. 3 tablespoons = _____ teaspoons

22. 2 cups = _____ ounces

23. 8 ounces = _____ pint(s)

24. 2 glasses = _____ pint(s)

25. 2 ounces = _____ tablespoons

26. 1/4 cup = _____ ounces

27. 3/4 cup = _____ ounces

28. 3 pints = _____ quart(s)

29. 6 teaspoons = _____ ounce(s)

30. 2 pints = _____ ounces

31. 1/2 teaspoon = _____ drops

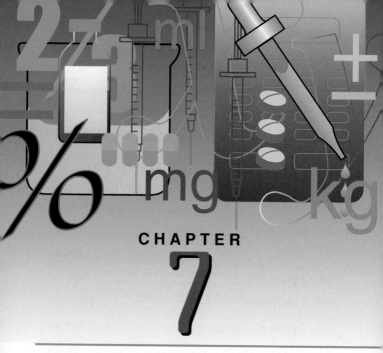

CHAPTER

7

Approximate Equivalents and System Conversions

120

• Convert approximate equivalents between the metric
  and apothecary systems and household measurements.

In the previous chapter, you learned how to change
units from one measurement to another *within the
same system*. Frequently, you will have to *convert
between systems*. When converting, you work with
approximate equivalents because exact measurements across different systems are not possible. A
common example of such a discrepancy is between
the metric and apothecary systems. For example, a
medication label will indicate 5 grains, and its
equivalent dosage may be written as 300 mg or 325
mg. Both dosages are correct; the equivalent values
are approximate.

Because you will have to calculate dosages for
medications between the apothecary and metric systems and household measurements, two tables of
equivalent values have been provided. You must
memorize the equivalents found in Tables 7.1 and
7.2. Remember when calculating dosages,
division is carried out two decimal places and
decimals are rounded off to ensure accuracy
(Appendix B).

The metric and English household equivalents
for length are rarely used for drug dosage calculations but can be used when applying a paste,
cream, or ointment that needs to cover a
certain area. However, both are used for linear
measurements—e.g., to measure wound size, head
circumference, abdominal girth, and height
(Table 7.2).

TABLE 7.1 Volume and Weight Equivalents

METRIC SYSTEM	APOTHECARY SYSTEM	HOUSEHOLD MEASUREMENTS
Volume		
—	1 minim	1 drop
1 milliliter	15–16 minims	15–16 drops
4–5 milliliters	1 dram (60 minims)	1 teaspoon (60 gtts)
15 milliliters	4 drams (3–4 teaspoons)	1 tablespoon (1/2 ounce)
30 milliliters	1 ounce (8 drams)	2 tablespoons (1 ounce)
180 milliliters	6 ounces	1 teacup
240 milliliters	8 ounces	1 glass/ measuring cup
500 milliliters	1 pint	1 pint (16 ounces)
1,000 milliliters (1 liter)	1 quart	1 quart (32 ounces)
	2 pints	1 quart
	4 quarts	1 gallon
Weight		
0.60–0.65 milligrams	gr 1/100	—
0.5 milligrams	gr 1/120	—
0.4 milligrams	gr 1/150	—
0.3 milligrams	gr 1/200	—
0.2 milligrams	gr 1/300	—
1,000 micro- grams	gr 1/60	—
1 milligram (1,000 microgram)	gr 1/60	—
4 milligrams	gr 1/15	—
6 milligrams	gr 1/10	—
10 milligrams	gr 1/6	—
15 milligrams	gr 1/4	—

TABLE 7.1 Volume and Weight Equivalents (continued)

METRIC SYSTEM	APOTHECARY SYSTEM	HOUSEHOLD MEASUREMENTS
60–65 milligrams	1 grain	—
1 gram (1,000 mg)	15 grains	—
4–5 grams	1 dram	—
15 grams	4 drams	—
30 grams	8 drams	1 ounce
454 grams	12 ounces	1 pound
1 kilogram (1,000 grams)		2.2 pounds

Dosage Problems for Medications: Converting Between Systems

Whenever the physician orders a drug in a unit that *is in a different system from the drug that is available,* convert to the available system. You want to work in the system of the drug that you have on hand.

TABLE 7.2 Linear Equivalents for the Household and Metric Systems

HOUSEHOLD	METRIC
1 inch	2.5 centimeters 25 millimeters
12 inches (1 foot)	30 centimeters
39.4 inches (1 yard + 3.4 inches)	1 meter

> **RULE: Whenever the desired and available drug doses are in two different systems, you would: choose the equivalent value and solve for *x*. Always change the desired quantity to the available quantity.**

Example: Give 12 drams of a drug that is available in mL.

- Select the approximate equivalent value and convert to the system that you have available.

Change 12 drams to mL (mL are available).

- Choose the equivalent value.

8 drams = 30 mL

- Complete the proportion. Write down *what you know.* A colon format is used here.

8 drams : 30 mL :: 12 drams : *x*

$8x = 360$

- Solve for *x:*

$8x = 360$

$$\frac{8^1 x}{8_1} = \frac{360^{45}}{8_1} \quad x = 45 \text{ mL}$$

Answer: 45 mL

Example: Give gr 1/4 of a drug that is available in mg.

- Select the approximate equivalent value and convert to the system that you have available.

    Change gr 1/4 to mg
    (mg are available).

- Choose the equivalent value.

    60 mg = 1 grain

- Complete the proportion. Write down *what you know.* A colon format is used here.

    60 mg : 1 gr :: x mg : gr 1/4

    $x = 60 \times 1/4$

- Solve for x:

    $${}^{15}\cancel{60} \times \frac{1}{\cancel{4}_1} = 15 \quad x = 15 \text{ mg}$$

    Answer: 15 mg

PRACTICE PROBLEMS

Complete the following. Solve for x or the unknown by using a fraction or colon format.

1. 12 f℥ = _____ mL

2. 0.3 mL = _____ L

3. 3 mL = _____ m

4. 45 mg = _____ gr

5. 2 tsp = _____ mL

6. 30 kg = _____ lbs

Complete the following. Solve for *x* or the unknown by using a fraction or colon format.

7. gr 1/200 = ____ mg

8. 3 pt = _____ mL

9. 6 ʒ = _____ g

10. 300 mcg = ____ mg

11. 30 mL = ____ oz

12. 4 tbs = _____ mL

13. 6 mg = _____ gr

14. 3 g = _____ gr

15. 1 L = _____ qt

16. 2 qts = _____ L

17. 2.2 lb = ____ kg

18. s̄s oz = _____ ʒ

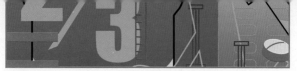

End of Chapter Review

Complete the following. Solve for *x* by using a fraction or colon format.

1. A child who weighs 55 pounds weighs _____ kg.

2. Two (2) ounces of Metamucil powder is equivalent to _____ g.

3. A patient is restricted to four 8-ounce glasses of water/day or _____ mL/day.

4. A patient's abdominal wound measures 10 cm in diameter. The nurse knows this is equivalent to _____ inch(es).

5. A child was prescribed 1 fluidram of cough syrup, four times a day, as needed. The child's mother administered _____ tsp each time the medication was given.

6. The nurse administered aspirin gr v. She knew this was equivalent to _____ mg.

7. The nurse instilled 3 minims of an eye drop into the patient's right eye, three times per day. The nurse knew that 3 minims was equal to _____ gtt.

8. The physician prescribed 0.4 mg of atropine sulfate to be administered intramuscularly. The medication was labeled in gr/mL. The nurse knew to look for an ampule labeled _____ gr/mL.

9. A patient was to take 2 tbsp of milk of magnesia. Because a medicine cup was available, he poured the milk of magnesia up to the _____ dram calibration line.

10. A 20-kg child was ordered a drug (15 mcg/kg of body weight). The child should receive _____ mcg or _____ mg.

11. A woman was prescribed 60 mg of a daily vitamin. Her cumulative monthly dose (30 days) would be about _____ g.

12. A patient who takes 1 tbsp of Kayexalate four times per day would be receiving a daily dose equivalent to _____ oz.

13. A patient takes a 500-mg tablet three to four times per day. He is advised not to exceed a daily dose of 3 g or _____ tablets.

14. A patient is to receive 250 mg of a liquid medication, three times daily. The medicine is available in oral suspension, 250 mg/5 mL. The nurse would give _____ tsp or _____ ℥.

15. An elderly patient is prescribed 30 mg of a drug as a single bedtime dose. The drug is available as a syrup at a concentration of 10 mg/5 mL. The nurse would give _____ mL or _____ tsp.

16. A patient is to receive a 200-mg tablet every 12 hours. The tablet is available in 200-mg quantities. The patient would receive _____ g per day.

17. A child is prescribed a 250-mg tablet every 6 hours. The nurse gives two tablets, four times a day. Each tablet would be _____ mg for a daily total dosage of _____ g.

18. A renal patient, whose daily fluid intake is restricted to 1,200 mL/day, is prescribed eight oral medications, three times daily. The nurse

restricts the water needed for swallowing the medications so the patient can have fluids with his meals. The patient is allowed 5 oz of water, three times a day with his medications. Therefore, the patient has _____ mL with his drugs.

19. A physician prescribes 0.5 mL of a drug/kg of body weight for a patient who weighs 120 pounds. The nurse would give _____ mL.

20. Tylenol liquid is available as 325 mg/5 mL. A patient who is prescribed 650 mg would be given _____ tsp.

21. A patient is to receive 10 mg of a drug available as 40 mg/2 mL. The nurse would give _____ mL.

22. A physician prescribes 0.3 mg of a drug, twice daily. The medication is available in 0.15-mg tablets. The nurse would give _____ tablets each dose, equivalent to _____ mg daily.

End of Unit 2 Review

Convert each item to its equivalent value.

1. 0.080 g = _____ mg

2. 3.2 liters = _____ mL

3. 1,500 mcg = _____ mg

4. 0.125 mg = _____ mcg

5. 20 kg = _____ g

6. 5 mg = _____ g

7. $3\overline{ss}$ = _____ dram(s)

8. 30 minims = _____ dram(s)

9. 15 grains = _____ dram(s)

10. 1/2 quart = _____ ounces

11. 3 pints = _____ quart(s)

12. 8 drams = _____ ounce(s)

13. 1 tbs = _____ tsp

14. 6 tsp = _____ ounce(s)

15. 1 teacup = _____ ounces

16. 2 tbs = _____ ounce(s)

17. gr $\overline{ss}$ = _____ mg

18. 30 grams = _____ ounce(s)

19. 1 oz = _____ mL

20. 1 gr = _____ mg

21. 3 tsp = _____ mL

22. 20 kg = _____ pounds

23. gr 1/150 = _____ mg

24. 0.3 mg = _____ gr

25. 1.8 oz = _____ mL

26. 20 mL = _____ tsp

27. 8.5 g = _____ mg

28. 950 mg = _____ g

29. 15 mg = _____ gr

30. 6 mg = _____ mcg

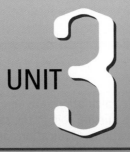

UNIT 3

Dosage Calculations

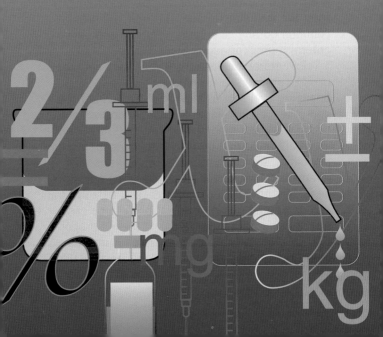

Accurate dosage calculations are an essential component of the nursing role in the safe administration of medications. Medications are prescribed by their generic (official) name or trade (brand) name and are usually packaged in an average unit dose. Oral medications contain a solid concentration of drug, per quantity of one (e.g., Tylenol gr x). Liquid medications contain a specific amount of drug, usually gram weight, dissolved in solution (e.g., mL); for example, Demerol @ 50 mg/mL or Vistaril @ 25 mg/5 mL. Medication orders refer to drug dosages, so calculations will be necessary if a dosage prescribed is different (system and/or unit of measurement) from the available dosage. This unit will present common dosage calculations for oral and parenteral routes for adults and children.

Parenteral medications (IM, SC) are packaged in vials, ampules, and premeasured syringes. Some are available as a single-dose preparation and others are available in multiple doses. Dosages usually range from 1 mL to 3 mL. Some drugs are measured in units (e.g., heparin, insulin, penicillin), some are found in solutions as mEq (grams per 1 mL of solution), and others need to be reconstituted from a powder (e.g., Kefzol). Oral and parenteral dosage calculations can be completed using a fraction format, ratio and proportion, or Dimensional Analysis, which is introduced in Chapter 9. Intravenous solutions are available in various quantities (e.g., 250 mL, 500 mL, 1,000 mL). Critical care intravenous solutions are prescribed in smaller quantities and administered via an electronic pump. Examples of these dosage calculations can be found in Chapter 12.

All medications come packaged and are clearly labeled. Each label must contain specific information as outlined in Chapter 8. Remember: you should never prepare or administer any medication that is not clearly labeled.

Infants and children cannot receive the same dose of medication as adults because a child's physiologic immaturity influences how a drug is absorbed, excreted, distributed, and used. Therefore, pediatric dosages are based on age, body weight, or body surface area. If you are going to give pediatric drugs, you must become familiar with the rules for calculating pediatric dosages, which can be found in Chapter 15. Refer to Appendix I for nursing concerns for pediatric drug administration. The older adult also responds differently to the metabolism of medications. See Appendix K for nursing concerns for geriatric drug administration. Appendix J suggests nursing considerations for critical care drug administration.

Medication Labels

LEARNING OBJECTIVES

After completing this chapter, you should be able to:

- Identify a drug's generic and trade name on a medication label.
- Identify drug dosage strength, form, and quantity on a medication label.
- Interpret drug administration requirements and precautions on a medication label.
- Interpret drug manufacturing information on a medication label.

- Interpret drug reconstitution or mixing directions on a medication label.
- Recognize when drug dosage calculations, including equivalent conversions, are necessary; for example, when the prescribed dose is different than the available dose.
- List the six patient rights specific to drug administration.

To prepare the correct medication that is prescribed, you must be able to accurately read a drug label and be familiar with major key points presented in this chapter. Several drug labels will be depicted as examples and sample drug problems will be presented.

Reading and Interpreting a Drug Label

Some labels are easy to read because they contain a limited amount of information; for example, labels for unit dose preparation where each tablet or capsule is separately packaged. This is the most common type of label that you will see in a hospital setting. Other labels indicate multiple tablets or capsules, with the dosage of each drug clearly visible.

Some solid preparations are available in a liquid solution. Frequently drugs are ordered in a unit of measure different from what is available. Mathematical conversions will be required, which will be covered in detail in the chapters that follow.

- **Drug name:** Medications are prescribed by their trade or generic name. Drug labels contain *essential and comprehensive* information for the safe administration of medications.
  - **Generic or official name:** The chemical name given by the company that initially manufactures the drug. It appears in smaller letters, sometimes in parentheses, under the brand name. A drug has only one chemical name, but it may have many different trade names. As a cost-control effort, some insurance companies are now requiring that pharmacists offer a generic brand first, unless contraindicated by the physician.
  - **Trade, brand, or proprietary name:** The commercial or marketing name that the pharmaceutical company gives a drug. It is printed in bold, large, or capital letters on the label. The ® identifies manufacturer ownership. The drug may be manufactured and marketed by several companies, each using its own trade name.
- **Drug dosage and strength:** The amount of drug available by weight per unit of measure (e.g., Nexium, 40-mg capsules; Demerol, 50 mg/mL). Sometimes the dosage is expressed in two systems (e.g., Nitrostat 0.4 mg [1/150 gr]). Dosage strength is indicated in a solid form (e.g., g, mg, mEq, mcg), in a solid form within a liquid (e.g., mg/mL), in solutions (e.g., 1:1,000), in units (e.g., 1,000 U/mL), or in other preparations such as ointments or patches.

  Examine the drug label for multiple doses of *Coreg* (see Figure 8.1). Each of the 100 tablets contain 12.5 mg of the solid drug prochlorperazine. The usual dose of 12.5 mg/day to 25 mg/day means

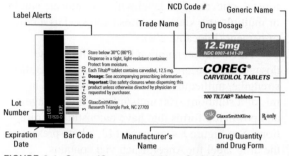

Label Alerts

NCD Code #   Generic Name

Trade Name   Drug Dosage

Store below 30°C (86°F).
Dispense in a tight, light-resistant container.
Protect from moisture.
Each Tiltab® tablet contains carvedilol, 12.5 mg.
Dosage: See accompanying prescribing information.
Important: Use safety closures when dispensing this
product unless otherwise directed by physician or
requested by purchaser.

GlaxoSmithKline
Research Triangle Park, NC 27709

12.5mg
NDC 0007-4141-20

COREG®
CARVEDILOL TABLETS

100 TILTAB® Tablets

gsk GlaxoSmithKline   R only

Lot
Number

Expiration   Bar Code   Manufacturer's   Drug Quantity
Date   Name   and Drug Form

FIGURE 8.1 Coreg (Courtesy of GlaxoSmithKline,
Philadelphia, PA).

that a patient may receive 1 to 2 or more tablets
daily.

- **Drug form:** The form in which the drug is prepared by the manufacturer; for example, tablets,
  capsules, injectables, oral suspensions, supposito-
  ries, ointments, and patches. Some drugs are prepared in several forms. The drug label may also
  indicate specific characteristics of the drug's form;
  for example, sustained release (SR), controlled
  release (CR) or long acting (LA).

- **Drug quantity:** The total amount of the drug in the
  container (e.g., 100 tablets, 30 capsules, 10 mL) or
  the total amount of liquid available after reconstitution (e.g., 5 mL, 50 mL). See Figure 8.3 on page
  142, which shows the drug label for Augmentin.
  When the powder is reconstituted with 47 mL of
  water, each 5 mL of liquid contains 200 mg of
  the drug.

- **Drug administration:** The route indicated on the
  label, such as oral, sublingual, IM, IV, SC, rectal,

topical, otic, etc. The label will also indicate single- or multiple-use vials, or doses expressed as a ratio or percent (lidocaine 2%).

Parenteral preparation labels will indicate dosages in a variety of ways: percentage and ratio strengths, milliequivalents (number of grams in 1 mL of a solution), 100 units/mL (insulin dosages), and powdered forms that have reconstitution directions. See Figure 8.4 on page 142, which presents the drug label for Ancef. Each vial contains approximately 330 mg/mL (IM use) after the addition of 2 mL of sterile water.

- **Drug reconstitution or mixing:** As shown in Figures 8.3 and 8.4 (page 142), the directions for mixing and reconstitution are clear on the drug labels. *Always follow these directions* to ensure the accuracy of drug preparation.

- **Drug manufacturing information:** By federal law, drug labels must contain the following information: **manufacturer name, expiration or volume date, control numbers, a National Drug Code (NDC) number** that is different for every drug, **a bar code** (used for a drug distribution system), and a code identifying one of two official national lists of approved drugs: **USP (United States Pharmacopeia) and NF (National Formulary).** These are identified in Figure 8.1 (page 139).

- **Drug precautions**: Drug labels also contain precautions about storage and protection from light. For example: Septra tablets (store at 59°F to 77°F in a dry place), heparin (store at controlled room temperature [59°F to 86°F]), promethazine HCl (protect from light and keep covered in the carton until time of use), and Coreg (protect from moisture).

Expiration dates indicate the last date that the drug should be used. *Never give a drug beyond its expiration date!*

- **Patient's rights:** As a nurse, you must honor the six rights of patients: right person, right drug, right dosage, right route, right time, and the right to refuse.

PRACTICE PROBLEMS

Fill in the blanks for the following questions, referring to the medication labels for Requip (Figure 8.2), Augmentin (Figure 8.3), and Ancef (Figure 8.4).

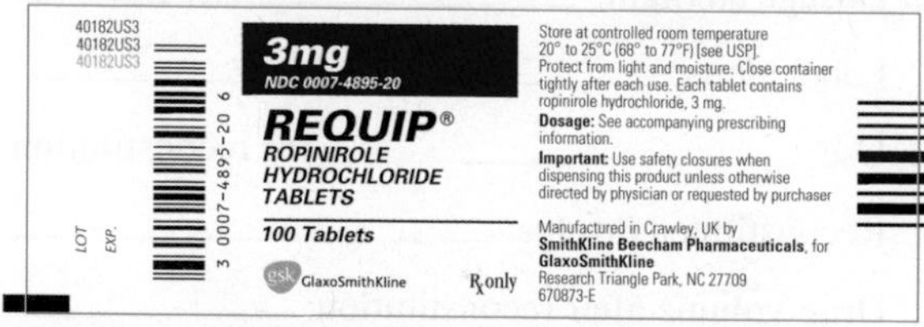

FIGURE 8.2 Requip (Courtesy of GlaxoSmithKline, Philadelphia, PA).

1. Generic name: _____

2. NDC number: _____

3. Dosage strength: _____

4. Drug quantity: _____

5. Drug form: _____

6. Label alerts: _____

7. Trade name: _____

8. Manufacturer: _____

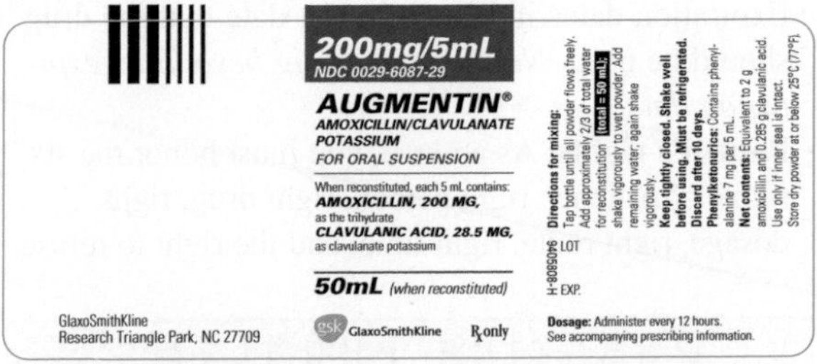

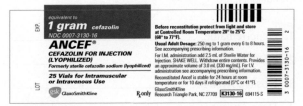

FIGURE 8.3 Augmentin (Courtesy of GlaxoSmithKline, Philadelphia, PA).

1. Generic name: _____

2. Dosage strength: _____

3. Label alerts: _____

4. Use _____ for reconstitution

5. Reconstituted dosage: _____

6. Drug volume after reconstitution: _____

FIGURE 8.4 Ancef (Courtesy of GlaxoSmithKline, Philadelphia, PA).

1. Proprietary name: _____

2. Identify two routes of administration: _____

   and _____

3. Reconstitute with: _____

4. Approximate dose/mL after reconstituting:

_____

5. Usual adult dose: _____

6. Label alerts: _____

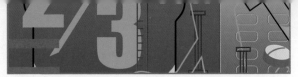

End of Chapter Review

Answer each question by referring to the specific drug labels presented in Figures 8.5, 8.6, 8.7, 8.8, and 8.9.

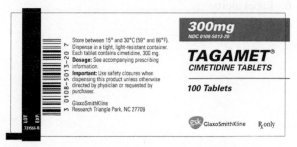

FIGURE 8.5 Tagamet (Courtesy of GlaxoSmithKline, Philadelphia, PA).

1. A physician prescribed 300 milligrams of Tagamet four times a day. The nurse would administer _____ tablet(s) for each dose. The patient would receive _____ milligrams of Tagamet in 24 hours.

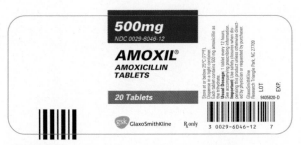

FIGURE 8.6 Amoxil (Courtesy of GlaxoSmithKline, Philadelphia, PA).

2. A patient is to receive 2 grams of amoxicillin (Amoxil) every 24 hours for 10 days. The medication is given every 6 hours. The patient would receive _____ milligrams or _____ grams for each dose.

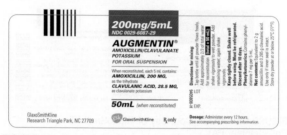

FIGURE 8.7 Augmentin (Courtesy of GlaxoSmithKline, Philadelphia, PA).

3. A physician prescribed 100 milligrams of Augmentin every 8 hours for a 3-year-old. The medication comes in a powder for an oral suspension, with a concentration of 200 mg/5 mL. The nurse would administer _____ mL for each dose. The child would receive _____ mg and _____ mL in 24 hours.

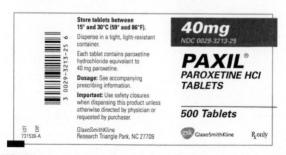

FIGURE 8.8 Paxil (Courtesy of GlaxoSmithKline, Philadelphia, PA).

4. A physician prescribed 40 milligrams of Paxil twice a day. The patient would receive _____ tablet(s) per dose and _____ milligrams per day.

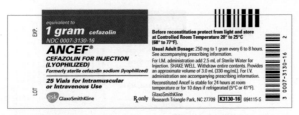

FIGURE 8.9 Ancef (Courtesy of GlaxoSmithKline, Philadelphia, PA).

5. A physician prescribed 1 gram of Ancef, intra-muscularly, every 8 hours. The nurse would need to mix _____ vial(s) for each dose.

6. A patient is prescribed 500 mg of Ancef intra-muscularly, immediately. The nurse would recon-stitute the vial of Ancef with _____ mL of sterile water for injection.

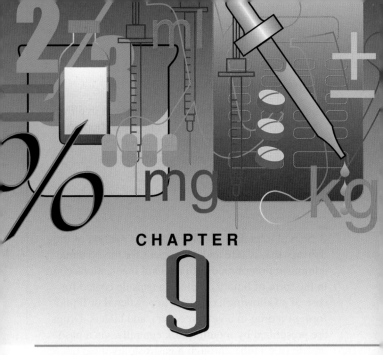

Oral Dosage Calculations

LEARNING OBJECTIVES

After completing this chapter, you should be able to:

- Apply the Formula Method to calculate drug dosage problems.
- Use Dimensional Analysis to solve drug dosage problems.
- Solve dosage calculations for medications in the same system using either ratio and proportion, the Formula Method, or Dimensional Analysis.

- Solve dosage calculations for medications in different systems using either ratio and proportion, the Formula Method, or Dimensional Analysis.
- Understand the rationales for critical thinking checks.

The oral route is a simple, economic method of drug delivery that is safe and convenient for the systemic administration of medications. Oral medications come in the form of liquids, caplets (a capsule coated for ease of swallowing), capsules (a powdered or liquid form of a drug in a gelatin cover), and tablets. Drugs are prescribed by mouth (p.o.), enterally, via a nasogastric (n.g.) tube, through a gastrostomy tube, or through a percutaneous endoscopic gastrostomy (P.E.G.) tube. Most tablets, capsules, and caplets come in the dosage prescribed, or the prescription requires giving more than one pill, breaking a scored tablet in half or quarters, or crushing and/or mixing a dose when swallowing is difficult. Enteric-coated tablets (a coating that promotes intestinal rather than gastric absorption) and sustained-release capsules (absorbed over time) should be taken whole. See Figure 9.1 for an example of an oral drug preparation.

Calculating Oral Dosages

When medications are prescribed and available in the same system (e.g., metric) and the same unit of

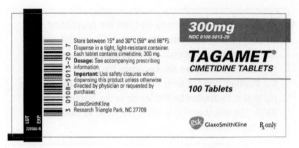

FIGURE 9.1   Tagamet (Courtesy of GlaxoSmithKline, Philadelphia, PA).

size (e.g., mg), dosage calculations are easy. When the prescribed or desired dosage is different from what is available or what "you have," you must convert to the same system (usually metric) and the same units (the smaller the better) before calculating dosages.

When calculating oral dosages, you can use either ratio and proportion, the Formula Method, or Dimensional Analysis. You have learned how to use ratio and proportion in Chapter 4. The Formula Method and Dimensional Analysis will be presented here.

The Formula Method

The Formula Method is a quick approach for solving dosage calculations. Always use critical thinking checks to make sure your answer is logical. Sometimes it will be necessary to convert between and within systems before calculating the dosage. Examples will be provided after the RULE.

> RULE: To apply the Formula Method: the *prescribed* amount of drug becomes the *desired (D)* amount and the numerator of the fraction; the drug that is *available*, the amount that *you have (H),* becomes the denominator of the fraction; and the drug form (tablet, mL) is the *quantity (Q)* that is multiplied by the terms in the fraction labeled (D/H). The unknown (*x*) is what you need to calculate to give the medication.

$$\frac{\text{D (desired amount)}}{\text{H (have available)}} \times \text{Q (quantity)}$$

$$= x \text{ (amount to give)}$$

$$\left[\frac{\text{D}}{\text{H}} \times \text{Q} = x \right]$$

When calculating dosages for drugs in solid form, the drug amount is identified per one tablet or capsule. When the drug is in a liquid form, the medication (mcg, mg, mEq) is dissolved in the solution (mL, oz). *The symbol R_x is used throughout this book to indicate "desired amount."*

Dimensional Analysis

Dimensional Analysis is a process commonly referred to as the *factor method* because drug dosages are considered *factors* and calculations are solved using a *factor method.* The unit of measure is the drug form being calculated (mL, tablet, capsule, etc.). *A fraction format is used for this formula!* As with the other formulas, always convert prior to calculating dosages.

> **RULE: To apply the Dimensional Analysis formula: follow the steps in the example given below.**

Example: Give 500 mg of a drug twice daily. The drug is available as 0.25 g/tablet.

- On the left side of the equation, list the desired unit of measure first, followed by an equals sign. The desired unit is the form that you want to give (tablet, capsule, mL).

$$x \text{ tab} =$$

- Look at what you have available (0.25 g/tablet). This information is placed to the right of the equals sign. The numerator of the new fraction must be the same unit of measure as the desired unit currently to the left of the equals sign (x tab). The denominator is the available drug amount (0.25 g).

$$x \text{ tab} = \frac{1 \text{ tablet}}{0.25 \text{ g}}$$

- The first fraction is called the "starting factor," and it is followed by the multiplication symbol ($\times$) to set up the proportion format.

$$x \text{ tab} = \frac{1 \text{ tablet}}{0.25 \text{ g}} \times$$

- Look at what is ordered and add additional factors. The numerator of the second fraction must match the unit of measure in the first denominator.

Therefore, the unit of measure "grams" must be in the numerator of the second fraction. Because 500 mg is the desired dose, 500 mg is changed to 0.5 g. You can place a 1 under 0.5 g to complete the fraction without changing the fraction's value.

$$x \text{ tab} = \frac{1 \text{ tablet}}{0.25 \text{ g}} \times \frac{0.5 \text{ g}}{1}$$

• Cancel the opposite and matching units of measure in the denominator and numerator. The remaining measure (tablet) is what is desired. Complete the mathematical calculations.

$$x \text{ tab} = \frac{1 \text{ tablet}}{0.25} \times \frac{0.5}{1} = \frac{0.5}{0.25} = 2$$

Answer: 2 tablets

Dosage Calculations for Medications in the Same System and the Same Unit of Measurement

> **RULE:** Whenever the desired and available drug doses are different but in the same system and same unit of measurement, you can use one of the following three methods to calculate dosages.

Example: R_x: 0.250 mg
             Have: 0.125-mg tablet
             Give: _____ tablet(s)

The sample problem will be solved using all three formulas.

Use Ratio and Proportion

0.125 mg : 1 tablet :: 0.250 mg : x

$0.125x = 0.250$

$x = \dfrac{0.250}{0.125} = 2$ tablets

Use the Formula Method

$\dfrac{D}{H} \times Q = x$

$\dfrac{0.250 \text{ mg}}{0.125 \text{ mg}} = 0.250 \div 0.125 = 2$

$2 \times (1 \text{ tablet}) = 2$ tablets

Use Dimensional Analysis

$x \text{ tab} = \dfrac{1 \text{ tab}}{0.125 \text{ mg}} \times \dfrac{0.250 \text{ mg}}{1}$

$x \text{ tab} = \dfrac{1}{0.125} \times \dfrac{0.250}{1} = \dfrac{0.250}{0.125} = \dfrac{250}{125} = 2$ tablets

---

Example: R_x: gr 1/2 p.r.n.

           Have: gr 1/4/tablet

           Give: _____ tablet(s)

Use Ratio and Proportion

gr 1/4 : 1 tablet :: gr 1/2 : x tablet

$1/4 \, x = 1/2$

$x = \dfrac{1/2}{1/4} = \dfrac{1}{2} \times \dfrac{4}{1} = 2$ tablets

Use the Formula Method

$$\frac{D}{H} \times Q = x$$

$$\frac{\text{gr } 1/2}{\text{gr } 1/4} = \frac{1}{2_1} \times \frac{4^2}{1} = \frac{2}{1} = 2$$

$2 \times (1 \text{ tablet}) = 2 \text{ tablets}$

Use Dimensional Analysis

$$x \text{ tab} = \frac{1 \text{ tablet}}{\text{gr } 1/4} \times \frac{\text{gr } 1/2}{1}$$

$$x \text{ tab} = \frac{1}{1/4} \times \frac{1/2}{1} \times \frac{1/2}{1/4} = \frac{1}{2} \times \frac{4}{1} = 2 \text{ tablets}$$

Example: R_x: 100 mg
                Have: 20 mg/5 mL
                Give: _____ mL

Use Ratio and Proportion

20 mg : 5 mL :: 100 mg : x

$20x = 500$

$$x = \frac{500}{20} = \frac{50}{2} = 25 \text{ mL}$$

Use the Formula Method

$$\frac{D}{H} \times Q = x$$

$$\frac{100 \text{ mg}}{20 \text{ mg}} = 100 \div 20 = 5$$

$5 \times (5 \text{ mL}) = 25 \text{ mL}$

Use Dimensional Analysis

$$x \text{ mL} = \frac{5 \text{ mL}}{20 \text{ mg}} \times \frac{100 \text{ mg}}{1}$$

$$x \text{ mL} = \frac{5}{20} \times \frac{100}{1} = 25 \text{ mL}$$

Dosage Calculations for Medications in the Same System but With Different Units of Measurement

> **RULE: Whenever the desired and available drug doses are in the same system but different units of measurement, you would: convert to like units, change to the smaller unit, and use one of three methods to calculate dosages.**

Example: R$_x$:   4 grams daily
            Have: 500 mg/tablet
            Give: _____ tablet(s)

Convert to Like Units: To convert 4 g to mg, move the decimal point (4.0 g) three places to the right: 4.000.

Then 4 g = 4,000 mg

Use Ratio and Proportion
500 mg : 1 tablet :: 4,000 mg : x

500 x = 4,000

$$x = \frac{4,000}{500} = \frac{40}{5} = 8 \text{ tablets}$$

Use the Formula Method

$$\frac{D}{H} \times Q = x$$

$$\frac{4,000 \text{ mg}}{500 \text{ mg}} = \frac{4,000}{500} = \frac{40}{5} = 8 \text{ tablets}$$

Use Dimensional Analysis

$$x \text{ tab} = \frac{1 \text{ tablet}}{500 \text{ mg}} \times \frac{4,000 \text{ mg}}{1}$$

$$x \text{ tab} = \frac{1}{500} \times \frac{4,000}{1} = \frac{4,000}{500} = \frac{40}{5} = 8 \text{ tablets}$$

Example:	R_x: 1.2 grams in 2 divided doses
	Have: 600 mg/tablet
	Give: _____ tablet(s)
Convert to Like Units:	To convert 1.2 g to mg, move the decimal point (1.2 g) three places to the right: 1.200.
	Then 1.2 g = 1,200 mg

Use Ratio and Proportion

600 mg : 1 tablet :: 1,200 mg : x

$600 x = 1,200$

$$x = \frac{1,200}{600} = 2 \text{ tablets in 2 divided doses or 1 tablet}$$
each dose

Use the Formula Method

$$\frac{D}{H} \times Q = x$$

$$\frac{1,200 \text{ mg}}{600 \text{ mg}} = 1,200 \div 600 = 2$$

2 × quantity (1 tablet) = 2 tablets in 2 divided doses or 1 tablet each dose

Use Dimensional Analysis

$$x \text{ tab} = \frac{1 \text{ tab}}{600 \text{ mg}} \times \frac{1,200 \text{ mg}}{1}$$

$$x \text{ tab} = \frac{1}{600} \times \frac{1,200}{1} = \frac{1,200}{600} = \frac{12}{6} = 2 \text{ tablets in}$$

divided doses or 1 tablet each dose

Dosage Calculations for Medications in Different Systems

> **RULE: Whenever the desired and available drug doses are in different systems, you would: convert to the same system (use available system), select the equivalent value, write down what you know in a fraction or ratio format, and use one of three methods to calculate dosages.**

Example:

R$_x$: Morphine sulfate grain 1/4
Have: Morphine sulfate 10-mg tablets
Give: _____ tablet(s)

Convert to Same System:

Milligrams are *available*.
Change gr 1/4 to mg

Equivalent: 1 grain = 60 mg

Complete the Proportion: 1 grain : 60 mg :: 1/4 grain : x mg

$$1 \times x = \frac{1}{4} \times 60$$

Solve for x: $\quad 1x = \frac{1}{4} \times 60$

$$1x = 15$$

$$x = 15 \text{ mg}$$

Use Ratio and Proportion

10 mg : 1 tablet :: 15 mg : x

$$10x = 15$$

$$x = \frac{15}{10} = 1\frac{1}{2} \text{ tablets}$$

Use the Formula Method

$$\frac{D}{H} \times Q = x$$

$$\frac{15 \text{ mg}}{10 \text{ mg}} = 15 \div 10 = 1.5$$

$$1.5 \times 1 \text{ tablet} = 1.5 \text{ or } 1\frac{1}{2} \text{ tablets}$$

Use Dimensional Analysis

$$x \text{ tablets} = \frac{1 \text{ tab}}{10 \text{ mg}} \times \frac{15 \text{ mg}}{1}$$

$$x \text{ tablets} = \frac{1}{10} \times \frac{15}{1} = \frac{15}{10} = 1\frac{1}{2} \text{ tablets}$$

PRACTICE PROBLEMS

1. R_x: 160 mg daily
   Have: 40-mg tablets
   Give _____ tablet(s).

2. R_x: 1500 mg
   Have: 500 mg/5 mL
   Give _____ mL.

3. R_x: 150 mg
   Have: 300-mg tablets
   Give _____ tablet(s).

4. R_x: 20 mg
   Have: 10 mg/5 mL
   Give _____ mL.

5. R_x: 7.5 mg t.i.d.
   Have: 2.5-mg tablets
   Give _____ tablet(s), t.i.d.

6. R_x: 100 mg every 4 to 6 hours, as needed
   Have: 50-mg tablets
   Give _____ tablet(s) for each dose.

7. R_x: 75 mg
   Have: elixir 15 mg/mL
   Give _____ mL.

8. R_x: 25 mg
   Have: 50-mg tablets
   Give _____ tablet(s).

9. R$_x$: 0.030 mg

   Have: 0.05-mg tablets

   Give _____ tablet(s).

10. R$_x$: 10 mg

    Have: 2.5-mg tablets

    Give _____ tablet(s).

11. R$_x$: 75 mg t.i.d.

    Have: 25-mg tablets

    Give _____ tablet(s).

12. R$_x$: 300 mg

    Have: 125 mg/5 mL

    Give _____ mL.

13. R$_x$: 0.75 grams

    Have: syrup labeled 250 mg/5 mL

    Give _____ mL.

14. R$_x$: 0.5 grams

    Have: syrup labeled 250 mg/5 mL

    Give _____ mL.

15. R$_x$: 4 grams to be taken in four equally
    divided portions

    Have: 500-mg tablets

    Give _____ tablet(s) each dose.

Critical Thinking Check:

Refer to question 15. If 5 grams were ordered in five divided doses, does it seem logical that one 500-mg tablet would be given? _____ **Yes or No?**

16. R$_x$: 0.25 g

    Have: elixir labeled 100 mg/5 mL

    Give _____ mL.

17. R$_x$: 2.0 grams daily

    Have: 250-mg tablets

    Give _____ tablet(s) each day.

18. R$_x$: 0.5 g every 8 hours

    Have: an oral suspension labeled 250 mg/
    teaspoon

    Give _____ mL.

Critical Thinking Check:

Refer to question 18. Since the suspension was ordered every 8 hours, does it seem logical that the patient should be awakened during the night for his medication? _____ **Yes or No?**

---

19. R$_x$: 0.30 grams daily

    Have: 100-mg capsules

    Give _____ tablet(s) each day.

20. R$_x$: 10 mg

    Have: 2.5-mg tablets

    Give _____ tablet(s).

21. R$_x$: 0.8 g

    Have: 400-mg tablets

    Give _____ tablet(s).

22. A mediation is on hand in syrup (2 mg/mL). The prescribed dose is 3 teaspoons. Give _____ mL, which would be equal to _____ mg.

23. A drug is on hand in a liquid as 250 mg/5 mL. The initial dose of 125 mg for 3 days requires giving _____ teaspoon(s) each day for a total of _____ mL over 3 days.

24. A medication is on hand in a transdermal patch containing 0.0015 grams. The system delivers 0.5 mg over 72 hours. After 72 hours, grains _____ remain.

25. R_X: gr x as an elixir

    Have: 160 mg/teaspoon

    Give _____ mL.

26. R_X: 1.2 mg

    Have: gr 1/100

    Give _____ tablet(s).

27. R_X: 20 mg

    Have: gr 1/6 tablets

    Give _____ tablet(s).

28. R_X: gr v

    Have: 300-mg tablets

    Give _____ tablet(s).

29. R_X: 50-mg oral suspension

    Have: 25 mg/5 mL

    Give _____ teaspoons.

30. R_X: gr 1/100 tablets

    Have: 0.6-mg tablets

    Give _____ tablet(s).

31. R$_x$:   suspension 500

    Have: 250 mg/5 mL

    Give _____ mL = _____ teaspoons.

32. R$_x$:   20 mEq, q.i.d.

    Have: elixir available as 6.7 mEq/5 mL

    Give _____ mL or _____ ounce(s).

33. R$_x$:   gr i $\overline{ss}$

    Have: 50-mg capsules

    Give _____ capsule(s). The dose is
    approximate.

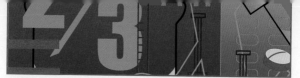

End of Chapter Review

Solve the following problems:

1. R$_X$:   30 mg daily
   Have: 10-mg tablets
   Give _____ tablet(s).

2. R$_X$:   300 mg
   Have: 100-mg tablets
   Give _____ tablet(s).

3. R$_X$:   1.5 grams daily
   Have: liquid labeled 250 mg/5 mL
   Give _____ mL.

4. R$_X$:   0.2 grams
   Have: 50-mg tablets
   Give _____ tablet(s).

5. R$_X$:   grain 1/200
   Have: 0.3-mg tablets
   Give _____ tablet(s).

6. R$_X$:   grain 1/2
   Have: 15-mg tablets
   Give _____ tablet(s)..

7. R$_X$:   20 grams
   Have: 30 grams in 45 mL
   Give _____ ounce(s).

8. R$_X$:   grain 1/150
   Have: 0.4-mg tablets
   Give _____ tablet(s).

9. R: grain 1/4

    Have: oral solution labeled 10 mg/5 mL

    Give _____ mL.

10. R: 0.1 gram

    Have: 100-mg tablets

    Give _____ tablet(s).

11. R: gr 1/4 four times a day

    Have: 15-mg tablets

    Give _____ tablet(s) per dose for a total
    of _____ tablet(s) daily.

12. R: 10 mg daily for 2 weeks

    Have: 2.5-mg tablets

    Give _____ tablets daily, equally divided
    over 6 hours.

Critical Thinking Check:

Refer to question 12. If the drug was ordered
q.i.d. rather than every 6 hours, would you
expect the patient to receive the same number
of pills in 24 hours? _____ **Yes or No?**

---

13. R: 5 mg

    Have: 1.25-mg tablets

    Give _____ tablet(s).

14. R: 500,000 units q.i.d.

    Have: 100,000 U/mL

    Give _____ teaspoon(s) or _____ dram(s).

15. R_x: 500 mg

    Have: 0.25 g/5 mL

    Give _____ mL or _____ teaspoon(s).

Critical Thinking Check:

Refer to question 15. Does it seem logical that 1 gram of the drug could also be prescribed based on the available dosage? _____ **Yes or No?**

---

16. R_x: 1.5 grams daily in three equal doses, for hypertension. The nurse would give _____ mg tablet(s), three times a day.

17. R_x: 2.4 grams daily for rheumatoid arthritis

    Have: 600 mg tablets

    Give _____ tablet(s) a day.

18. R_x: 30 mg

    Have: gr 1/4 tablet

    Give _____ tablet(s).

19. R_x: gr v

    Have: 300-mg tablets

    Give _____ tablet(s).

CHAPTER 10

Parenteral Dosage Calculations

LEARNING OBJECTIVES

After completing this chapter, you should be able to:

- Define the term *parenteral* as it refers to medication delivery.
- Distinguish between ampules, vials, and different types of syringes used for parenteral drug administration.
- Read the calibrations on a syringe.

• Calculate parenteral medication dosages using ratio and proportion, the Formula Method, and Dimensional Analysis.

T he term *parenteral* refers to any route of drug delivery other than gastrointestinal. Parenteral commonly refers to the injection of drugs via a needle and syringe into body tissues (IM—into a muscle, SC—into subcutaneous tissue) and into body fluids (IV—into a vein or an infusion). Remember: needle *precautions should always be followed* when administering parenteral medications.

The parenteral route is recommended if a medication needs to be rapidly administered or would be ineffectively absorbed in the gastrointestinal tract or take too long to become effective. Parenteral drugs are administered in the form of sterile liquid preparations (powder forms are reconstituted) and should absorb easily without causing tissue irritation.

Packaging and Types of Syringes

Parenteral medications are most commonly supplied in liquid or solution form and packaged in ampules (small, glass, sealed containers), vials (small, glass or plastic bottles with a rubber tip), and prefilled cartridges and syringes that contain a single drug dose. There are three kinds of syringes: hypodermic, tuberculin, and insulin. Insulin syringes will be presented

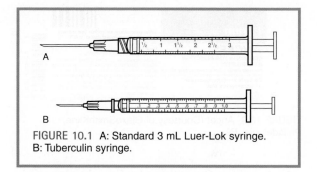

FIGURE 10.1 A: Standard 3 mL Luer-Lok syringe.
B: Tuberculin syringe.

later in Chapter 13. See Figure 10.1 for an example of a standard, 3-mL, Luer-Lok hypodermic syringe and a 1-mL tuberculin syringe.

Syringes have three parts: a barrel with mL calibrations, a plunger, and a tip. Luer-Lok syringes have a tip that syringe-specific needles twist into; non–Luer-Lok syringes have a tip that needles slip into. Some syringes have a safety glide (covers needle after use), while others are needleless (intravenous use).

The 3-mL syringe is marked in 0.1-mL increments with longer lines indicating 0.5 mL and 1.0 mL. Markings on the 1-mL tuberculin syringe can be found in tenths (0.1 mL) and hundredths (0.01 mL). It is essential that you read the calibrations accurately so the correct amount of medication can be given. When checking the liquid medication in the syringe, remember to always (a) hold the syringe *at eye level* and (b) use the *top of the black ring* to measure the correct amount.

Most injectable medications are given in a 3-mL syringe unless the dosage can easily be measured in

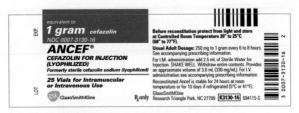

FIGURE 10.2 Ancef (Courtesy of GlaxoSmithKline, Philadelphia, PA).

a 1-mL syringe. Quantities <1 mL can be given in a tuberculin syringe. See Figures 10.2 and 10.3 for examples of labels for two different parenteral drug preparations.

Pediatric parenteral medications are most commonly given via the subcutaneous and intramuscular routes. Dosage amount is limited to 1 mL per site for those under 5 years of age, and dosages are usually measured using a tuberculin syringe. Children ages 6–12 can be given up to 2 mL of solution per site; the volume limit for adults is 3 mL per site. Pediatric dosages will be covered in more detail in Chapter 15.

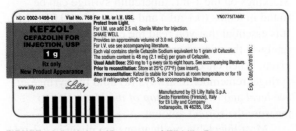

FIGURE 10.3 Kefzol (Courtesy of Eli Lilly Company, Indianapolis, Indiana).

To calculate parenteral dosage problems, follow the same rules that you used for oral dosage calculations. The Formula Method is recommended whenever possible; ratio and proportion and Dimensional Analysis can also be used. Remember to follow the guidelines regarding patient age, size, and special considerations before administering parenteral needs.

Dosage Calculations for Medications in the Same System and the Same Unit of Measurement

> **RULE: Whenever the desired and available drug doses are different but in the same system and the same unit of measurement, you would: use one of three methods to calculate dosages.**

Example: R_x: 1.0 mg
               Have: 5.0 mg/mL
               Give: _____ mL

Use Ratio and Proportion

5.0 mg : 1 mL :: 1.0 mg : x mL

$5x = 1.0$

$x = \dfrac{1}{5} = 0.2$ mL

Answer: 0.2 mL

Use the Formula Method

$$\frac{D}{H} \times Q = x$$

$$\frac{1.0 \text{ mg}}{5.0 \text{ mg}} = \frac{1}{5}$$

$$\frac{1}{5} \times 1 \text{ mL} = 0.2 \text{ mL}$$

Answer: 0.2 mL

Use Dimensional Analysis

$$x \text{ mL} = \frac{1 \text{ mL}}{5.0 \text{ mg}} \times \frac{1.0 \text{ mg}}{1}$$

$$x \text{ mL} = \frac{1}{5} \times \frac{1}{1} = \frac{1}{5} = 0.2 \text{ mL}$$

Answer: 0.2 mL

Example: R_x: 300 mg
           Have: 150 mg/mL
           Give: _____ mL

Use Ratio and Proportion

150 mg : 1.0 mL :: 300 mg : x mL

$$150x = 300$$

$$x = \frac{300}{150} = 2 \text{ mL}$$

Answer: 2 mL

Use the Formula Method

$$\frac{D}{H} \times Q = x$$

$$\frac{300 \text{ mg}}{150 \text{ mg}} = \frac{2}{1}$$

$$\frac{2}{1} \times 1 \text{ mL} = 2 \text{ mL}$$

Answer: 2 mL

Use Dimensional Analysis

$$x \text{ mL} = \frac{1 \text{ mL}}{150 \text{ mg}} \times \frac{300 \text{ mg}}{1} =$$

$$x \text{ mL} = \frac{1}{150} \times \frac{300}{1} = \frac{300}{150} = 2 \text{ mL}$$

Answer: 2 mL

Example: R$_x$:   35 mg
Have: 50 mg/mL
Give: _____ mL

Use Ratio and Proportion

50 mg : 1 mL :: 35 mg : x

$$50x = 35$$

$$x = \frac{35}{50} = \frac{7}{10} = 0.7 \text{ mL}$$

Answer: 0.7 mL

Use the Formula Method

$$\frac{D}{H} \times Q = x$$

$$\frac{35 \text{ mg}}{50 \text{ mg}} = \frac{7}{10}$$

$$\frac{7}{10} \times \text{quantity (1 mL)} = 0.7 \text{ mL}$$

Answer: 0.7 mL

Use Dimensional Analysis

$$x \text{ mL} = \frac{1 \text{ mL}}{50 \text{ mg}} \times \frac{30 \text{ mg}}{1} =$$

$$x \text{ mL} = \frac{1}{50} \times \frac{30}{1} = \frac{3}{5} = 0.7 \text{ mL}$$

Answer: 0.7 mL

Dosage Calculations for Medications in the Same System but Having Different Units of Measurement

> **RULE: Whenever the desired and available drug doses are in the same system but of different units of measurement, you would: convert to like units, change to the smaller unit, and use one of three methods to calculate dosages.**

Example: R_x: 0.25 mg
            Have: 500 mcg/2 mL
            Give: _____ mL

Convert   To convert 0.25 mg to mcg, move the
to Like   decimal point (0.25 mg) three places
Units: to the right 0.250. Then 0.25 mg =
             250 mcg.

Use Ratio and Proportion
500 mcg : 2 mL :: 250 mcg : x mL

$500x = 500$

$x = \dfrac{500}{500} = 1$ mL

                                   Answer: 1 mL

Use the Formula Method
$\dfrac{D}{H} \times Q = x$

$\dfrac{250 \text{ mcg}}{500 \text{ mcg}} = \dfrac{1}{2}$

$\dfrac{1}{2} \times$ quantity (2 mL) = 1 mL

                                   Answer: 1 mL

Use Dimensional Analysis
$x \text{ mL} = \dfrac{2 \text{ mL}}{500 \text{ mcg}} \times \dfrac{250 \text{ mcg}}{1}$

$x \text{ mL} = \dfrac{2}{500} \times \dfrac{250}{1} = \dfrac{500}{500} = 1$ mL

                                   Answer: 1 mL

Dosage Calculations for Medications in Different Systems

> **RULE:** Whenever the desired and available drug dosages are in different systems, you would: convert to the same system (use available system), select the equivalent value, write down what you know in a fraction or ratio format, and use ratio and proportion to solve for *x*. Use one of three methods to calculate dosages.

Example: R_x: gr $\overline{\text{iss}}$ IM, b.i.d.
Have: 60 mg/mL
Give: _____ mL, b.i.d.

Equivalent: 1 grain = 60 milligrams

Complete the Proportion: 1 grain : 60 mg :: $1\frac{1}{2}$ grains : x mg

$$1 \times x = 1\frac{1}{2} \times 60$$

Solve for x: $1x = 1\frac{1}{2} \times 60$

$$1x = \frac{3}{2_1} \times \cancel{60}^{30}$$

$$x = 90 \text{ mg}$$

Use Ratio and Proportion

60 mg : 1 mL :: 90 mg : x mL

$$60x = 90$$

$$x = \frac{90}{60} = 1.5 \text{ mL}$$

Answer: 1.5 mL

Use the Formula Method

$$\frac{D}{H} \times Q = x$$

$$\frac{90 \text{ mg}}{60 \text{ mg}} = \frac{3}{2}$$

$$\frac{3}{2} \times 1 \text{ mL} = 1\frac{1}{2} \text{ mL}$$

Answer: $1\frac{1}{2}$ mL

Use Dimensional Analysis

$$x \text{ mL} = \frac{1 \text{ mL}}{60 \text{ mg}} \times \frac{90 \text{ mg}}{1} =$$

$$x \text{ mL} = \frac{1}{60} \times \frac{90}{1} = \frac{90}{60} = 1.5 \text{ mL}$$

Answer: 1.5 mL

Penicillin

Penicillin is one of a limited number of medications that is available in units/mL as well as mg/mL. Insulin (covered in Chapter 13) and heparin (covered in Chapter 14) are two other common medications that you will need to become familiar with. When calculating dosages for penicillin, you can use ratio and proportion, the Formula Method, or Dimensional Analysis.

> **RULE: To prepare penicillin for injection, you would: check units to be given and use one of three methods to calculate dosages.**

Example: A patient is prescribed 300,000 units of penicillin G procaine to be administered q12h. Penicillin G procaine is available as 600,000 units/1.2 mL.

Use Ratio and Proportion

600,000 U : 1.2 mL :: 300,000 : x mL

600,000x = 300,000 × 1.2

600,000x = 360,000

$x = \dfrac{360,000}{600,000} = \dfrac{36}{60} = \dfrac{6}{10} = 0.6$ mL

Answer: 0.6 mL

Use the Formula Method

$\dfrac{D}{H} \times Q = x$

$\dfrac{300,000 \text{ U}}{600,000} = \dfrac{300,000}{600,000} = \dfrac{3}{6} = \dfrac{1}{2}$

$\dfrac{1}{2} \times 1.2$ mL = 0.6 mL

Answer: 0.6 mL

Use Dimensional Analysis

x mL $= \dfrac{1.2 \text{ mL}}{600,000} \times \dfrac{300,000}{1}$

x mL $= \dfrac{1.2}{6} \times \dfrac{3}{1} = \dfrac{3.6}{6} = 0.6$ mL

Answer: 0.6 mL

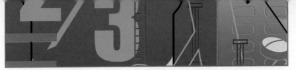

End of Chapter Review

1. Give 0.002 grams of a drug, IM, per day, for 5 days, for severe intestinal malabsorption. The injection was on hand as 1.0 mg/mL. The nurse would give _____ mL a day for 5 days.

2. Give 60 mg of a diuretic IM in three equally divided doses every 8 hours for 2 days. The drug is available for injection as 10 mg/mL. The nurse should give _____ mL every 8 hours.

3. Give 0.3 grams of a drug that is available as 100 mg/mL for injection. The nurse would give _____ mL.

4. Give 10 mg of a drug that is available as 5 mg/mL. The nurse should draw up _____ mL.

5. Give 4 mg of a drug that is available as 5 mg/mL. The nurse should give _____ mL.

6. Give 125 mg of a drug, IV, to be added into 100 mL NSS and hung as an intermittent infusion. The medication is available as 250 mg/ 5mL. The nurse would prepare _____ mL.

> ## Critical Thinking Check:
>
> If the available medication is twice the amount of drug prescribed, does it seem logical that half the quantity (mL) would be given? _____
> **Yes or No?**

7. Give 2 mg of a drug, IV, p.r.n., every 4 to 6 hours. The medication is available as 5 mg/mL. The nurse would give _____ mL every 3 to 4 hours as needed.

8. The physician requested that a patient receive 1.5 mg of a drug, IM, every 3 to 4 hours as needed for pain. The medication is available for injection as 2.0 mg/mL. The nurse would give _____ mL every 3 to 4 hours, p.r.n.

9. Give 35 mg, IM, of a drug that is available for injection as 50 mg/mL. The nurse would give _____ mL.

10. Give 6 mg of a drug, weekly. The medication is available as 2 mg/mL. The nurse would give _____ mL every week.

11. Give 3 mg, IM, of a drug preoperatively to induce drowsiness. The drug is available as 5 mg/mL. The nurse would give _____ mL.

12. Give 1 mg, IV, of a drug every 4 to 6 hours for analgesia. The drug is available as 4 mg/mL. The nurse would give _____ mL every 4 to 6 hours.

13. Give 30 mg, IV, of a diuretic. The drug is available as 40 mg/mL. The nurse would give _____ mL.

14. Give 0.5 mg of a medication that is available in a vial as grains 1/150 per 1.0 mL. The nurse would give _____ mL.

15. Give 50 mg of a medication that is available in vials containing grains i per mL. The nurse would give _____ mL.

16. Give grains 1/5, IM, every 4 to 6 hours for severe pain. The medication is available as 15 mg/mL. The nurse would give _____ mL, every 4 to 6 hours, as needed.

Critical Thinking Check:

Since the available medication strength (15 mg/mL) is a stronger drug concentration than the prescribed medication (gr. 1/5), does it seem logical that >1 mL would be given? _____ **Yes or No?**

17. Give 6 mg of a drug by IV push. The medication is available as 10 mg/mL for injection. The nurse would give _____ mL.

18. Give 0.15 mg IM of a drug that is available as 0.2 mg/mL. The nurse would give _____ mL.

19. Give 25 mg, IM, of a drug preoperatively. The drug is available as 100 mg/2 mL. The nurse would give _____ mL.

20. Give 50 mg, IV, q6h, of a drug that is available as 25 mg/mL. The nurse would give _____ mL.

21. Give 0.1 mg of a drug, IV, for a procedure requiring conscious sedation. The drug is available as 50 mcg/mL. The nurse would give _____ mL.

22. Give 500 mcg, IM, of a drug that is available as 1 mg/mL. The nurse would give _____ mL.

23. Give 30 mg, IV push, of a drug that is available as 20 mg/mL. The nurse would give _____ mL q4h.

Critical Thinking Check:

Does it seem logical that since a smaller dosage of drug/mL is available than the amount that is prescribed that the quantity given would be

---

24. Give 0.25 mg, IV, of a drug that is available as 250 mcg/mL. The nurse would give _____ mL q4 weeks.

25. Give 4 mg, IV, of a drug that is available as 2 mg/mL. The nurse would give _____ mL.

26. Give gr 1/4, q6h, of a drug that is available as 30 mg/mL. The nurse would give _____ mL.

27. Give 90 mg of a drug, IV, q6h, that is available as 120 mg/2 mL. Give _____ mL.

28. Give 0.05 mg of a drug that is available as 100 mcg/0.5 mL. Give _____ mL.

29. Give 0.4 g of a drug that is available as 500 mg/ 5 mL. Give _____ mL.

30. Give 250 mg of a drug that is available as 0.75 g/ 3 mL. Give _____ mL.

31. The physician prescribed Crysticillin 600,000 units, IM, as a single dose. Crysticillin is available in a 12-mL vial labeled 500,000 U/mL. The nurse would give _____ mL.

32. The physician prescribed 300,000 units of Bicillin, IM, q12h for 5 days. Bicillin is packaged as 600,000 U/mL. The nurse would give _____ mL.

33. The physician prescribed penicillin G potassium 125,000 U, IM, q12h. The medication is available in solution as 250,000 U/5 mL. The nurse would give _____ mL every 12 hours.

34. Penicillin G benzathine 1.2 million units was prescribed, IM, as a single injection. The drug is available as 300,000 U/mL. The nurse would give _____ mL.

Critical Thinking Check:

Would it seem logical to give a dosage of 1.2 M units as a single injection? _____ **Yes or No?**

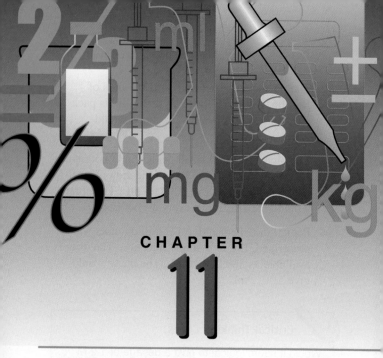

Intravenous Therapies

LEARNING OBJECTIVES

After completing this chapter, you should be able to:

- Explain the purpose of intravenous fluid therapy.
- Distinguish between continuous and intermittent fluid therapy.
- Distinguish between the purpose and types of volume-controlled and electronic volumetric pumps.

LEARNING OBJECTIVES (continued)

- Calculate milliliters per hour (mL/hr) for manual and electronic regulation.
- Calculate mL/hr for manual and electronic regulation when the infusion is *less than 1 hour.*
- Calculate drops per minute (gtt/min) using the Standard Formula and the Quick Formula.
- Calculate drops per minute using the Quick Formula with a constant factor.

Intravenous (IV) fluid therapy involves the administration of water, nutrients (e.g., dextrose, protein, fats, and vitamins), electrolytes (e.g., sodium, potassium, and chloride), blood products, and medications directly into a vein. Intravenous therapy, which can be *continuous or intermittent,* is used for fluid replacement or fluid maintenance to treat disorders like dehydration, malnutrition, and electrolyte imbalance.

Intravenous therapy is administered via an IV infusion set. The set consists of IV fluids in a sterile bag or bottle connected by IV tubing (includes a drip chamber with spike, one or more injection ports, a filter, and a slide or roller clamp) to the IV catheter in the patient's vein. The *primary* IV line is either a *peripheral* line, usually inserted into the arm or hand, or a *central* line, usually inserted into a large vein in the chest (subclavian) or neck (jugular). *Secondary* IV lines, also known as IV piggyback (IVPB) are used for intermittent, smaller quantity infusions (e.g., a medication in 50–100 mL of fluid) and are attached to the primary line through an injection port. A *peripherally inserted central catheter* (PICC line) is threaded into the superior vena cava through a vein in the arm.

IVPB solutions are usually given over 30–60 minutes. IVPB is always hung higher than the primary bag/bottle. *Remember:* the *greater* the height, the *greater* the pressure, the *faster* the rate of infusion! See Figure 11.1. If a piggyback medication

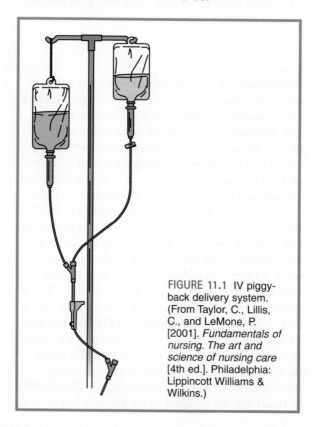

FIGURE 11.1 IV piggyback delivery system. (From Taylor, C., Lillis, C., and LeMone, P. [2001]. *Fundamentals of nursing. The art and science of nursing care* [4th ed.]. Philadelphia: Lippincott Williams & Wilkins.)

is to be given at the same time as the primary infusion, the bag/bottle is hung at the same height and the set-up is referred to as a *Tandem Set-Up*. Smaller quantities of solution (100–150 mL) and medications can be given via a burette chamber. These volume-controlled sets (Buretrol, Soluset, Volutrol) are frequently used for pediatric doses (see Chapter 15, Fig. 15.2).

Electronic Infusion Devices

Electronic infusion devices are used when small amounts of fluids/medications must be given over a strictly regulated period of time (usually used in pediatrics and critical care situations). These *are not gravity dependent!* There are several that you need to learn to use.

IV fluids are regulated by electronic volumetric pumps, syringe pumps, patient-controlled analgesia (PCA) devices and a balloon device used in home care. The *infusion pump* consistently exerts forced pressure against the resistance of the tubing or the fluid at a preselected rate. A pump improves the accuracy of delivering a set quantity; however, pumps can be dangerous because they continue to infuse even in the presence of infiltration or phlebitis. A *syringe pump* (a syringe filled with medication attached to a pump) regulates medications that must be given at a very low rate over a short period of time (5–20 minutes). A *PCA pump,* used by patients to self-medicate (pushing a control button), delivers a set amount of an IV narcotic contained in a prefilled syringe, within specified time periods, that are programmed into the pump. As a safety measure, there is a time interval when no medication can be delivered even if the patient pushes the button. The RN is responsible for the PCA loading dose, the narcotic injector vial, and the pump setting.

Intravenous Fluids

A physician's order for intravenous fluid therapy *must include* the type, quantity of solution, the time period for administration, and in some institutions or areas (pediatrics), the milliliters per hour. The physician's order is usually written as mL/hr to be infused (flow rate). The flow rate is regulated either manually by straight gravity, by volume control, or via an electronic infusion device.

Intravenous fluids are prepared in bags or bottles and the quantity of solution ranges from 50 mL to 1,000 mL. Solutions are clearly labeled.

Standard abbreviations are used for the type and concentration of solutions. Numbers refer to the percentage of the solution strength. Review the abbreviations in Table 11.1 and interpret the following sample physician orders, which must include solution name, quantity, added meds, and infusion rate and time.

- Administer 1,000 mL of D5W at 125 mL/hr.
- Administer 1,000 mL of 0.9% NSS every 12 hours for 2 days.
- Administer 500 mL of D10W at 83 mL/hr.
- Administer 100 mL of RL over 4 hours at 25 mL/hr.

TABLE 11.1 Commonly Prescribed Intravenous Fluids

FLUIDS	ABBREVIATIONS
0.9% Sodium chloride solution	NSS
0.45% Sodium chloride solution	1/2 NSS
0.25% Sodium chloride solution	1/4 NSS
5% Dextrose in water	5% D/W
	D5W
10% Dextrose in water	10% D/W
	D10W
5% Dextrose in 0.45% sodium chloride solution	D5 1/2
Dextrose with Ringer's lactate solution	D/RL
Ringer's solution	R
Lactated Ringer's solution	RL
Plasma volume expanders	
Dextran	
Albumin	
Hyperalimentation	
Total parenteral nutrition	TPN
Partial parenteral nutrition	PPN
Fat emulsions	
Intralipid	

Intravenous Flow Rate

The flow rate of the IV solution, as it passes through the drip chamber, is determined by the drop factor (gtt/mL) of the tubing set. The drop factor of the tubing set varies by manufacturer. Macrodrip sets (10, 15, and 20 gtt/min) are larger than micro-drip sets (60 gtt/min), which contain a needle in the

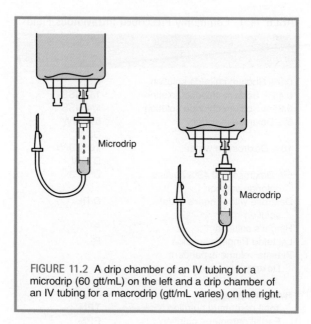

FIGURE 11.2 A drip chamber of an IV tubing for a microdrip (60 gtt/mL) on the left and a drip chamber of an IV tubing for a macrodrip (gtt/mL varies) on the right.

chamber to make the drops smaller. See Figure 11.2 and Table 11.2.

The IV infusion flow rate is always prescribed by the physician. The nurse is responsible for regulating flow rate in a variety of ways:

- *Calculating* infusion time (total hours for infusion)
- *Calculating* milliliters per hour (mL/hr), especially when an infusion device is used
- *Calculating* drops per minute (gtt/min) for IV sets (drop factor of IV tubing is needed)
- *Regulating* the number of drops entering the drip chamber by using the roller clamp on the tubing to

TABLE 11.2 Common Drop Factors for IV Tubing Sets

Macrodrop	10 gtt/mL
	15 gtt/mL
	20 gttt/mL
Microdrop	60 gtt/mL

adjust the flow rate (count number of drops for 1 minute). Remember to always hold a watch up to the drip chamber, at *eye level,* to accurately count the drops!

- *Setting* the infusion rate for electronic regulation in mL/hr

Calculating Infusion Time

A simple one-step ratio (division) is all that is needed when total volume is known and mL/hr has been ordered. Use this formula:

$$\frac{\text{Total volume}}{\text{mL/hr}} = \text{infusion time (round off minutes to nearest whole number)}$$

Example: The patient is to receive 1,000 mL of D5W solution at 75 mL/hr.

$$\frac{1,000 \text{ mL}}{75 \text{ mL}} = 13 \text{ hours and 33 min}$$

Answer: 13 hours and 33 min

Occasionally, you will need to determine infusion time when mL/hr is not provided. Follow this rule:

> **RULE: To calculate infusion time when mL/hr is unknown, you would: convert gtt/min to mL/min, convert mL/min to mL/hr, and use this formula:**
>
> $$\frac{\text{total volume}}{\text{mL/hr}} = \text{infusion time (hr)}$$

Example:	The physician prescribed 1,000 mL of RL to run at 30 gtt/min, using a drop factor of 15 gtt/mL.
Convert gtt/min to mL/min:	15 gtt : 1 mL :: 30 gtt : x mL
	$15 \times x = 1 \times 30$
	$15x = 30$
	$x = 2$ mL/min
Convert mL/min to mL/hr:	2 mL/min $\times$ 60 min = 120 mL/hr
Use:	$\dfrac{\text{total volume}}{\text{mL/hr}} = \text{infusion time}$
	$\dfrac{1,000 \text{ mL}}{120 \text{ mL/hr}} = 1,000 \div 120 = 8.3$ hours
Convert:	$\left(0.3 \text{ hr} = \dfrac{3}{10} \times 60 \text{ min} = 18 \text{ min}\right)$
	Answer: 8 hours and 18 min

Calculating Milliliters Per Hour for Manual or Electronic Regulation

To calculate mL/hr, all you need to know is the total volume to be infused over time. When a pump or controller is used, simply set the infusion rate at mL/hr to infuse the prescribed amount.

> ● **RULE: To calculate milliliters per hour, you would use one of three methods to calculate dosages.**

Example: A patient is to receive 1,000 mL of lactated Ringer's solution over a 6-hour period. The patient would receive _____ mL/hour.

Use Ratio and Proportion

1000 mL : 6 hr :: x mL : 1 hr

$6x = 1,000$

$x = 166.6$ mL/hr

Answer: 167 mL/hr

Use This Formula

$$\frac{\text{total volume (mL)}}{\text{total time (hours)}}$$

= milliliters per hour

$$\frac{1,000}{6} \text{ mL} = 166.6 \text{ mL/hr}$$

Round off to 167 mL/hr

Answer: 167 mL/hr

Use Dimensional Analysis

$$x \text{ mL/hr} = \frac{1,000 \text{ mL}}{6 \text{ hr}} = 166.6 \text{ mL}$$

Answer: 167 mL/hr

Calculating Milliliters Per Hour for Manual or Electronic Regulation When the Infusion is *Less Than 1 Hour*

When infusion time is less than 1 hour, total time in minutes needs to be used to solve for x (mL/hr).

> RULE: To calculate milliliters per hour when total time is less than 1 hour, you would use one of three methods to calculate dosages.

Example: A patient is to receive 1 gram of Rocephin in 50 mL of NSS over 30 minutes.

Use Ratio and Proportion

50 mL : 30 min :: x mL : 60 min (1 hr)

$30x = 3,000$

$$x = \frac{3,000}{30} = 100 \text{ mL/hr}$$

Answer: Set infusion rate at 100 mL/hr

Use This Formula

$$\frac{\text{total volume}}{\text{total time (min)}} = \frac{x \,(\text{mL/hr})}{60 \text{ min}}$$

$$\frac{50 \text{ mL}}{30 \text{ min}} = \frac{x \,(\text{mL})}{60 \text{ min}}$$

$$30x = 3,000$$

$$x = \frac{3,000}{30}$$

$$x = 100 \text{ mL/hr}$$

Answer: Set infusion rate at 100 mL/hr

Use Dimensional Analysis

$$x \text{ mL} = \frac{50 \text{ mL}}{30 \text{ min}} \times \frac{60 \text{ min}}{1}$$

$$x \text{ mL} = \frac{50}{30} \times \frac{60}{1} = \frac{3,000}{30} = 100 \text{ mL}$$

Answer: Set infusion rate at 100 mL/hr

Calculating Drops Per Minute

To calculate drops per minute, you need three pieces of information:

- The *total volume* to be infused in mL
- The *drop factor* of the tubing you will use*
- The *total time* for the infusion, *in minutes or hours*

---

*Check tubing package—may be 10, 15, 20 (macrodrip), or 60 (microdrip) gtt/mL.

You can use three methods to calculate the flow rate in drops per minute: the *Standard Formula*, Dimensional Analysis, and the *Quick Formula*. The Quick Formula can be used when milliliters per hour (mL/hr) replaces total volume.

The Standard Formula

$$\chi = \frac{\text{total volume} \times \text{drop factor}}{\text{total time (minutes)}}$$

$$= \text{drops per minute (gtt/min)}$$

Example: Administer 1,000 mL of D5W every 8 hours. The drop factor is 15 gtt/mL.

Use the Standard Formula

$$\frac{\text{total volume} \times \text{drop factor}}{\text{total time (minutes)}}$$

$$= \text{gtt/min}$$

$$\frac{1,000 \text{ mL} \times 15}{480 \text{ min } (60 \times 8)} = \frac{15,000}{480}$$

$$= 31.25 \text{ gtt/min}$$

Round off to 31 gtt/min

Answer: 31 gtt/min

Use Dimensional Analysis

$$x \text{ gtt/min} = \frac{15 \text{ gtt}}{1 \text{ mL}} \times \frac{1,000 \text{ mL}}{480 \text{ min}}$$

$$x \text{ gtt/min} = \frac{15}{1} \times \frac{15,000}{480} = 31.25 \text{ gtt/min}$$

Answer: 31 gtt/min

Example: Administer 500 mL of 0.9% NSS over 6 hours. The drop factor is 20 gtt/mL.

Use the Standard Formula

$$\frac{\text{total volume} \times \text{drop factor}}{\text{total time (minutes)}}$$

$= \text{gtt/min}$

$$\frac{500 \text{ mL} \times 20}{360 \text{ min}} = \frac{10,000}{360}$$

$= 27.7 \text{ gtt/min}$

Round off to 28 gtt/min

Answer: 28 gtt/min

Use Dimensional Analysis

$$x \text{ gtt/min} = \frac{20 \text{ gtt}}{1 \text{ mL}} = \frac{500 \text{ mL}}{360 \text{ min}}$$

$$x \text{ gtt/min} = \frac{20}{1} \times \frac{500}{360} = \frac{10,000}{360} = 27.7 \text{ gtt/min}$$

Answer: 28 gtt/min

Example: Administer 500 mL of a 5% solution of normal serum albumin over 30 minutes. The drop factor is 10. Calculate the flow rate in gtt/min.

Use the Standard Formula

$$\frac{\text{total volume} \times \text{drop factor}}{\text{total time (minutes)}}$$

$= \text{gtt/min}$

$$= \frac{500 \text{ mL} \times 10 \text{ gtt/mL}}{30 \text{ min}} = \frac{5,000}{30}$$

$$= 166.6 \text{ gtt/min}$$

Answer: 167 gtt/min

Use Dimensional Analysis

$$x \text{ gtt/min} = \frac{10 \text{ gtt}}{1 \text{ mL}} \times \frac{500 \text{ mL}}{30 \text{ min}}$$

$$x \text{ gtt/min} = \frac{10}{1} \times \frac{500}{30} = \frac{5,000}{30} = 166.6 \text{ gtt/min}$$

Answer: 167 gtt/min

The Quick Formula

$$\frac{\text{milliliters per hour (mL/hr)} \times \text{drop factor}}{\text{time (60 min)}} = \text{gtt/min}$$

Using the Quick Formula requires that you know the volume (mL/hr), drop factor, and time in minutes. Frequently, the physician's order indicates total volume, not mL/hr. Therefore, you would need to use the following to get mL/hr:

$$\frac{\text{total volume (mL)}}{\text{total time (hours)}} = \text{mL/hr}$$

Example: Give 1,000 mL of a drug over 10 hours. The drop factor is 20.

Calculate mL/hr:
$$\frac{\text{total volume (mL)}}{\text{total time (hours)}} = \text{mL/hr}$$

$$\frac{1,000 \text{ mL}}{10} = 100 \text{ mL/hr}$$

Use Quick Formula:

$$\frac{mL/hr \times drop\ factor}{time\ (60\ minutes)} = gtt/min$$

$$\frac{100\ mL/hr \times 20}{60\ min} = \frac{2,000}{60}$$

$$= 33.33\ gtt/min$$

Round off to 33 gtt/min

Answer: 33 gtt/min

Example: Administer 250 mL of 0.45% NSS over 5 hours. The drop factor is 60 gtt/mL.

Calculate mL/hr:

$$\frac{total\ volume\ (mL)}{total\ time\ (hours)} = mL/hr$$

$$\frac{250\ mL}{5\ hours} = 50\ mL/hr$$

Use Quick Formula:

$$\frac{mL/hr \times drop\ factor}{time\ (60\ minutes)} = gtt/min$$

$$= \frac{50\ mL/hr \times 60\ gtt/mL*}{60\ min} = \frac{3,000}{60}$$

$$= 50\ gtt/min$$

Answer: 50 gtt/min

---

*Please note: When a microdrip is used with a drop factor of 60, the gtt/min will always equal the mL/hr. If the physician orders an IV to run at 75 mL/hr with a microdrip, then the gtt/min is 75; if 35 mL/hr, then the gtt/min is 35.

Constant Factors

Quick Formula With Constant Factor

$$\frac{\text{milliliters per hour (mL/hr)}}{\text{constant factor}} = \text{gtt/min}$$

The constant factor is derived from the drop factor (of the administration set) divided into the fixed time factor of 60 minutes. It can only be used with the time factor of 60 minutes. Because the drop factor of 60 is the same as 60 minutes, these numbers cancel themselves out. A constant factor of 1 can be used in the division to replace both of these numbers. Therefore, for this Quick Formula, you can use the constant factor (1) to replace 60 minutes and 60 gtt/mL.

Because 60 remains constant for this Quick Formula, you can calculate constant factors for other drop factors by dividing by 60. Therefore, when working with a drop factor of 10, you can use the constant factor of 6 (60 ÷ 10); 15 would equal a constant factor of 4 (60 ÷ 15), and 20 would equal a constant factor of 3 (60 ÷ 20).

Example: Administer 1,000 mL of RL over 10 hours. The drop factor is 15 gtt/mL.

Use the Quick Formula

Calculate $\dfrac{\text{total volume}}{\text{total hours}} = \text{milliliters per hour}$
mL/hr:

$$\frac{1,000 \text{ mL}}{10 \text{ hours}} = 100 \text{ mL/hr}$$

Use the Constant Factor

$$\frac{\text{mL/hr}}{\text{constant factor}} = \text{gtt/min}$$

$$\frac{100 \text{ mL/hr}}{4 \, (60 \div 15)} = 25 \text{ gtt/min}$$

Answer: 25 gtt/min

Use Dimensional Analysis With the Constant Factor

$$x \text{ gtt} = \frac{100 \text{ mL}}{4 \, (60 \div 15)} = 25 \text{ gtt/min}$$

Answer: 25 gtt/min

PRACTICE PROBLEMS

1. The physician prescribed 1,000 mL of RL to infuse over 12 hours. You would give _____ mL/hr.

Critical Thinking Check:

Does it seem logical that if 1,000 mL is to be infused over 12 hours that the hourly amount would be <100 mL? _____ **Yes or No?**

2. You are to give 500 mL of NSS over 4 hours. You would give _____ mL/hr.

3. Administer 800 mL of NSS over 10 hours. The drop factor is 20 gtt/mL. You would give _____ gtt/min.

4. You are to give 1,000 mL of 0.45% NSS to infuse over 6 hours. The drop factor is 15 gtt/mL. You would give _____ gtt/min.

5. Administer 500 mL of solution over 24 hours. The drop factor is 60 gtt/mL. You would give _____ gtt/min.

6. You are to give 600 mL of solution over 12 hours. The drop factor is 20 gtt/mL. You would give _____ gtt/min.

Critical Thinking Check:

Would you expect the rate of the infusion to be faster or slower if the drop factor was 15 gtt/mL instead of 20 gtt/mL? _____ **Faster or slower?**

---

7. The physician prescribed an IV of 100 mL of D5W to run at 100 mL/hr. The drop factor is 10. You would set the flow rate at _____ gtt/min.

8. The physician prescribed an IV of Ringer's lactate at 75 mL/hr. The drop factor is 15. You would administer _____ gtt/min.

9. The physician prescribed an IV of NSS to be run at 60 mL/hr. The drop factor is 20. You would run the IV at _____ gtt/min.

10. Give 50 mg of an antibiotic in 100 mL of D5W over 30 minutes. The drop factor is 15 drops = 1 mL. You would piggyback this medication into the main IV and set the drip rate at _____ gtt/min.

11. The physician prescribed an IV of 1,500 mL of Ringer's lactate solution to infuse over 20 hours. The drop factor is 15 gtt/mL. You would give _____ gtt/min.

12. Administer 1 gram of an antibiotic in 50 mL of D5W over 30 minutes. The drop factor is 10 gtt/mL. The nurse would give _____ gtt/min.

13. The physician prescribed an IV of 250 mL of D5 0.22% NSS to infuse over 10 hours. The drop factor is 60 gtt/min. The nurse would give _____ mL/hr and _____ gtt/min.

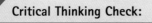

Critical Thinking Check:

If the drop factor of 60 is equal to the number of minutes in an hour (60), would it seem logical that the gtt/min would always equal the mL/hr? _____ **Yes or No?**

14. Administer 1 gram of an antibiotic in 100 mL of D5W to run over 30 minutes. The drop factor is 20 gtt/mL. You would give _____ gtt/min.

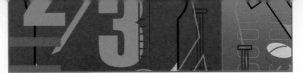

End of Chapter Review

Complete the following IV calculations:

1. To infuse 500 mL of solution over 8 hours, you would give _____ mL/hr.

2. Administer 1,000 mL over 10 hours. You would give _____ mL/hr.

3. To deliver 1,000 mL of D5 0.45% NSS over 4 hours, the nurse would have to administer _____ mL/hr.

4. To deliver 500 mL of D5W over a 6-hour period, the nurse would set the flow rate to deliver _____ mL/hr.

5. To deliver 250 mL of NSS over a 5-hour period, the nurse would set the flow rate to deliver _____ mL/hr.

6. A patient is to receive 500 mL of 0.45% NSS to run over 8 hours. The drop factor is 20 gtt/mL. The nurse would give _____ mL/hr.

7. Administer 1,000 mL of 0.9% NSS over 8 hours. The drop factor is 10 gtt/mL. The flow rate would be _____ gtt/min.

8. Administer 500 mL of D5W over a 12-hour period as KVO. The microdrip provides 60 gtt/mL. Use the Quick Formula with a constant factor. The flow rate would be _____ gtt/min.

9. To administer 1.0 liter of Ringer's lactate over 6 hours, you would give _____ mL/hr. The drop factor is 10 gtt/mL. The flow rate would be _____ gtt/min.

10. The physician prescribed 1,000 mL of D5W to infuse over 24 hours. With a drop factor of 15 gtt/mL, you would give _____ gtt/min. Use the Quick Formula with a constant factor.

11. The physician prescribed 1,000 mL of D5W 0.9% NSS to infuse at 75 mL/hr. The drop factor is 15 gtt/mL. You would give _____ gtt/min.

12. Ringer's lactate, 500 mL, is to infuse at 50 mL/hr. The drop factor is 10. You would set the rate at _____ gtt/min. Use the Quick Formula with a constant factor.

13. Administer 1,000 mL of RL at 50 mL/hr. The total infusion time would be _____ hours.

14. You are to give 500 mL of NSS at 40 mL/hr. The total infusion time would be _____ hours.

15. The physician prescribed 250 mL of D5W at 20 mL/hr. The total infusion time would be _____ hours.

16. The physician prescribed 100 mL of albumin to be absorbed over 2 hours. The drop factor is 15 gtt/mL. The nurse would run the IV at _____ gtt/min.

17. A patient is to receive 1,000 mL of NSS with 20,000 units of heparin over 24 hours. The drop factor is 60 gtt/mL. The nurse would give _____ gtt/min.

18. A patient is to receive 350 mg of an antibiotic in 150 mL of D5W over a 1-hour period of time. The drop factor is 15 gtt/mL. The nurse would give _____ gtt/min.

19. Administer 100 mL of an antibiotic solution via a volume control set over 60 minutes. The microdrip provides 60 gtt/mL. You would give _____ gtt/min.

20. The physician prescribed 500 mL of a 10% Intralipid solution to infuse over 4 hours. Using a controller, the nurse would set the rate at _____ mL/hr.

21. The patient is to receive 150 mg of a drug by slow IV push for status epilepticus. Dilantin is labeled 50 mg/mL. The nurse would give _____ mL over a 10-minute period.

22. The physician prescribed morphine sulfate 1 gram in 100 mL D5 NSS to infuse at 10 mg per hour. Calculate the flow rate in gtt/min. You would give _____ gtt/min using a microdrip.

23. A patient is to receive 1,200 mL of RL to run over 12 hours. The drop factor is 20 gtt/mL. The nurse would give _____ mL/hr and _____ gtt/min.

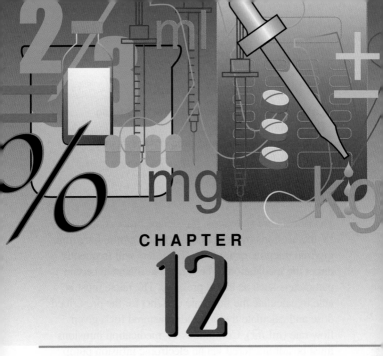

12

Intravenous Therapies: Critical-Care Applications

LEARNING OBJECTIVES

After completing this chapter, you should be able to:

- Calculate drug dosages and flow rates using either ratio and proportion or the Formula Method.
- Calculate drug dosages when the flow rate is known.

- Calculate drug dosages and flow rates using Dimensional Analysis.
- Calculate flow rates and drug dosages using constant factors.

In critical-care situations, physicians order continuous IV medications by drug dosage (mcg/kg/min, mcg/min, mg/min, mcg/hr, or mg/hr). The orders will frequently direct the medication to be titrated to maintain certain parameters such as blood pressure. The nurse must be able to calculate the flow rate (mL/hr) for the prescribed dose and calculate the dose administered for a given flow rate (mL/hr). Continuous IV medication infusions must be administered via an electronic infusion pump or controller. *Remember:* you must always know the safe dosage range of the medications you are administering before you begin the IV. Refer to Appendix J.

Calculating Drug Dosages and Flow Rates Using Either Ratio and Proportion or the Formula Method

> **RULE: To calculate flow rate (mL/hr) when the dosage is known, you would: convert to like units, convert to dose per minute if the drug is ordered by weight, and calculate mL/min or mL/hr using either ratio and proportion or the Formula Method.**

Example: Run Dobutamine 500 mg in 250 mL D5W at 5 mcg/kg/min to a patient

weighing 152 lbs. The electronic
infusion pump would be set
at _____ mL/hr.

Convert Change pounds to kg (2.2 lbs = 1 kg)
to Like 152 lbs ÷ 2.2 lbs/kg = 69.1 kg
Units:
         Change mg to mcg (1 mg = 1,000 mcg)
         500 mg × 1000 mcg = 500,000 mcg

Calculate 5 mcg/kg/min × 69.1 kg
mcg/min: = 345.5 mcg/min

Use Ratio and Proportion

345.5 mcg/min : x mL :: 500,000 mcg : 250 mL

500,000 mcg × x mL = 345.5 mcg/min × 250 mL

500,000x = 86,375

x = 0.173 mL/min

Calculate 0.173 mL/min × 60 min/hr
mL/hr: = 10.38 (10.4) mL/hr

Answer: 10.4 mL/hr

Use the Formula Method

$$\frac{D = \text{(desired amount in dose [mcg, mg, or units]/time [min or hr])}}{H = \text{(what you have available in the IV bag)}}$$

× Q (quantity in the IV bag) = x (mL/min or mL/hr)

Calculate $\dfrac{D}{H} \times Q = x$
mL/min
Using
Formula: $\dfrac{345.5 \text{ mcg/min}}{500,000 \text{ mcg}} \times 250 \text{ mL}$

         = 0.173 mL/min

Calculate	0.173 mL/min × 60 min/hr
mL/hr:	= 10.38 mL/hr

Answer: 10.4 mL/hr

Example: Amiodarone 900 mg in 500 mL D5W is prescribed to run at 0.5 mg/min. How many mL/hr should the patient receive?

Use Ratio and Proportion

900 mg : 500 mL :: 0.5 mg/min : x mL

$900x = 500 × 0.5$

$900x = \dfrac{250}{900} = \dfrac{25}{90} = 0.277 \ (0.278) \ \text{mL/min}$

Calculate	0.278 mL/min × 60 min/hr
mL/hr:	= 16.7 mL/hr

Answer: 16.7 mL/hr

Use the Formula Method

Calculate mg/min Using Formula:	$\dfrac{D}{H} × Q = x$
	$\dfrac{0.5 \ \text{mg/min}}{900 \ \text{mg}} × 500 \ \text{mL}$
	= 0.278 mL/min

Calculate	0.278 mL/min × 60 min/hr
mL/hr:	= 16.7 mL/hr

Answer: 16.7 mL/hr

> **RULE: To calculate dosage when the flow rate (mL/hr) is known, you would: convert to like units, calculate mL/min, and calculate dose (mcg, units, or mg/min) using the Formula Method. If drug is ordered by weight, calculate dose/kg/min.**

Example: | Dopamine 400 mg in 250 mL D5W has been increased to 10 mL/hr to maintain a systolic BP of 100 mm Hg in a patient weighing 115 lbs. How many mcg/kg/min should be infusing?

Convert to Like Units:

Change pounds to kg (2.2 pounds = 1 kg)
115 lbs ÷ 2.2 lbs = 52 kg

Change mg to mcg (1 mg = 1,000 mcg)
400 mg × 1,000 mcg = 400,000 mcg

Calculate mL/min:

10 mL/hr ÷ 60 min = 0.166 mL/min

Calculate mcg/min Using the Formula Method:

$$\frac{D}{H} \times Q = x$$

$$\frac{x \, \text{mcg/min}}{400,000 \, \text{mcg}} \times 250 \, \text{mL}$$

$$= 0.166 \, \text{mL/min}$$

Solve for x

$$\frac{x \, \text{mcg/min}}{400,000 \, \text{mcg}} \times 250 \, \text{mL} \div 250 \, \text{mL}$$

$$= 0.166 \, \text{mL/min} \div 250 \, \text{mL}$$

$$400,000 \times \frac{x \text{ mcg/min}}{400,000 \text{ mcg}}$$

$$= 0.00066 \times 400,000$$

$$x = 264 \text{ mcg/min}$$

Calculate mcg/kg/ min: 264 mcg/min ÷ 52 kg = 5.1 mcg/kg/min

Answer: 5.1 mcg/kg/min

Example: Fentanyl 4 mg in 250 mL D5W is titrated to 4 mL/hr to control pain. How many mcg/hr is currently infusing?

Convert to Like Units: (1,000 mcg = 1 mg)
1,000 mcg/mg × 4 mg = 4,000 mcg

Convert to mL/min: This step is not necessary because the dose is ordered in mcg/hr

Calculate mcg/hr Using Formula $$\frac{x \text{ mcg/hr}}{4,000 \text{ mcg}} \times 250 \text{ mL} = 4 \text{ mL/hr}$$

Solve for x

$$4,000 \text{ mcg} \times \frac{x \text{ mcg/hr}}{4,000 \text{ mcg}} \times 250 \text{ mL}$$

$$= 4 \text{ mL/hr} \times 4,000 \text{ mcg}$$

$$x \text{ mcg/hr} \times 250 = 16,000$$

$$x \text{ mcg/hr} \times 250 \div 250 = 16,000 \div 250$$

$$x = 64 \text{ mcg/hr}$$

Answer: 64 mcg/hr

Calculating Drug Dosages and Flow Rates Using Dimensional Analysis

> **RULE: To apply the Dimensional Analysis formula, follow the steps in the example below.**

Example: Run dobutamine 400 mg in 250 mL D5W at 12 mL/hr in a patient weighing 56 kg. You document that the patient is receiving _____ mcg/kg/min (dose).

- On the left side of the equation, list the unit of measure expressed in the dose

$$mcg/kg/min =$$

- Look at what you have available (400 mg/250 mL). This information is placed to the right of the equals sign. The numerator of the new fraction must be the same unit of measure as the desired unit currently to the left of the equals sign (mcg). Convert to like units (400 mg $\times$ 1,000 mcg/mg).

$$x \, mcg/kg/min = \frac{400,000 \, mcg}{250 \, mL}$$

- Look at what information is available and multiply by additional factors to cancel out units of measure to match the unit of measure on the left side of the equation. The numerator of the second fraction must match the unit of measure in the denominator of the first fraction. Therefore, the unit of measure (mL) must be in the numerator of the second fraction. Because the dose is administered in mL/hr, this becomes the second fraction.

$$x \text{ mcg/kg/min} = \frac{400,000 \text{ mcg}}{250 \text{ mL}} \times \frac{12 \text{ mL}}{\text{hr}}$$

- Since the dose on the left is expressed in minutes, an additional factor must be added to match the unit of measure in the denominator (hr). Hours must be converted to minutes by placing 1 hr/ 60 min next.

$$x \text{ mcg/kg/min} = \frac{400,000 \text{ mcg}}{250 \text{ mL}} \times \frac{12 \text{ mL}}{\text{hr}} \times \frac{1 \text{ hr}}{60 \text{ min}}$$

- The unit of measure on the left side of the equation contains kg in the denominator, so the right side of the equation must also contain kg in the denominator.

$$x \text{ mcg/kg/min} = \frac{\dfrac{400,000 \text{ mcg}}{250 \text{ mL}} \times \dfrac{12 \text{ mL}}{\text{hr}} \times \dfrac{1 \text{ hr}}{60 \text{ min}}}{56 \text{ kg}}$$

- Complete the mathematical calculations

$$x \text{ mcg/kg/min} = \frac{\dfrac{400,000 \text{ mcg}}{250 \text{ mL}} \times \dfrac{12 \text{ mL}}{\text{hr}} \times \dfrac{1 \text{ hr}}{60 \text{ min}}}{56 \text{ kg}}$$

Answer: 9 mL/hr

Example: Dobutamine 500 mg in 250 mL D5W is prescribed at 5 mcg/kg/min in a patient weighing 60 kg. You must set the pump at _____ mL/hr.

$$5 \text{ mcg/kg/min} = \cfrac{\cfrac{500{,}000 \text{ mcg}}{250 \text{ mL}} \times \cfrac{x \text{ mL}}{\text{hr}} \times \cfrac{1 \text{ hr}}{60 \text{ min}}}{60 \text{ kg}}$$

Answer: 9 mL/hr

Calculating Flow Rates and Drug Dosage Using Constant Factors

Constant factors can be used to recalculate changes in dosage or flow rates, providing the weight and the concentration of the drug infusion remain the same. This is carried out by solving the factors that remain the same (drug concentration, weight, and time) in a Dimensional Analysis equation and using that number (constant factor) to determine the missing component (dose or rate).

> RULE: To calculate the constant factor you would: calculate the amount of drug/mL in the IV bag in the units prescribed, then divide by kg (if ordered by weight), and then divide by 60 min (if ordered in minutes) or divide by 1 (if ordered in hours): *Dose unit (mcg, mg, etc.)/mL ÷ kg ÷ 60 min (or 1 if ordered in hours) = constant factors. Follow the guidelines listed below to use the constant factor.*

Using the Constant Factor

- The calculated constant factor is used to calculate either mL/hr or the dose.
- If the dose is known, divide the prescribed dose by the constant factor to calculate the desired flow rate (mL/hr).

• If the flow rate (mL/hr) is known, multiply the constant factor and the flow rate (mL/hr) to calculate the dose.

Example:	Primacor 50 mg in 250 mL D5W is prescribed to run at 0.375 mcg/kg/min in a patient weighing 58 kg. The pump should be set at _____ mL/hr.
Calculate the Amount of drug/mL:	50 mg ÷ 250 mL = 0.2 mg/mL Convert to mcg (1,000 mcg = 1 mg) 0.2 mg/mL × 1,000 mcg/mg = 200 mcg/mL
Divide by kg (if ordered by weight)	200 mcg/mL ÷ 58 kg = 3.45 mcg/kg/mL
Divide by 60 min (if ordered in minutes of by 1 hr (if ordered in hours)	3.45 mcg/kg/mL ÷ 60 min = 0.058 mcg/kg/mL in 1 min 0.058 is the **constant factor**
Calculate the Flow Rate (mL/hr):	Since the dose is known, divide the dose by the constant factor. 0.375 mcg/kg/min ÷ 0.058 mcg/kg/mL in a min = 6.5 mL/hr
	Answer: Set the pump at 6.5 mL/hr.

Example:	In the previous example, the physician orders the Primacor infusion to be decreased to 0.2 mcg/kg/min. The

patient's weight and the drug concentration remain the same. The patient should receive _____ mL/hr.

Calculate the Flow Rate Using the Constant Factor for This Patient:

Since the dose is known, divide the ordered dose by the constant factor. 0.2 mcg/kg/min ÷ 0.058 mcg/kg/mL in a min = 3.5 mL/min.

Answer: Reduce the infusion to 3.5 mL/min.

Example:

Esmolol 2,500 mg in 250 mL D5W is infusing at 21.6 mL/hr in a patient weighing 72 kg. How many mcg/kg/min should the patient receive?

Calculate the dose/mL:

2,500 mg ÷ 250 mL = 10 mg
Convert to mcg (1,000 mcg = 1 mg)
10 mg/mL × 1,000 mcg/mg
= 10,000 mcg/mL

Divide by kg (if ordered by weight)

10,000 mcg/mL ÷ 72 kg
= 138.8 mcg/kg/mL

Divide by 60 min (if ordered in minutes) or by 1 hr (if ordered in hours)

138.8 mcg/kg/mL in a minute
÷ 60 min = 2.31 mcg/kg/mL per min

Calculate the mcg/kg/min Using the Constant Factor for This Patient:

Since the mL/hr is known, multiply the flow rate (mL/hr) by the constant factor 2.31 mcg/kg/mL per min × 21.6 mL/hr = 50 mcg/kg/min

Answer: 50 mcg/kg/min

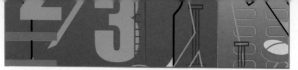

End of Chapter Review

1. The physician prescribes Tridil 50 mg in 250 mL D5W to start at 10 mcg/min to relieve chest pain. You would set the infusion pump at _____ mL/hr.

2. The nurse increases a lidocaine infusion of 2 g in 250 mL D5W to 30 mL/hr to control the patient's dysrhythmia. You would document that the patient is now receiving _____ mg/min.

3. The physician prescribes dopamine 400 mg in 250 mL D5W to start at 5 mcg/kg/min in a patient weighing 178 lbs. You would set the infusion pump at _____ mL/hr.

4. A 75-kg patient on a mechanical ventilator is sedated with Diprivan 1,000 mg in 100 mL at 10 mL/hr. You would document that the patient is receiving _____ mcg/kg/min.

5. The physician prescribes Ativan 250 mg in 250 mL to run at 3 mg/hr. You would set the infusion pump at _____ mL/hr.

6. The physician prescribes a continuous labetolol infusion to control hypertension. The label directs you to remove 90 mL from a 250-mL NSS bag and add 200 mg of labetolol. The labetolol vial has 5 mg/mL. You would add _____ mL of labetolol to the IV bag. The concentration of labetolol would be _____ mg/mL (remember to include the volume of the labetolol in the calculation of the total volume). In order to administer 1 mg/min, you would set the infusion pump at _____ mL/hr.

7. The physician prescribes a loading dose of procainamide 500 mg in 100 mL NSS over 30 minutes. The label reads procainamide 500 mg/mL. You would add _____ mL of procainamide to 100 mL NSS. You would set the infusion pump at _____ mL/hr to deliver this bolus. The loading dose is to be followed with a continuous infusion of procainamide 2 grams in 250 mL D5W to run at 2 mg/min. You would set the infusion pump at _____ mL/hr.

8. A patient is to receive a Cardizem bolus of 10 mg followed by a continuous infusion of Cardizem at 10 mg/hr. The Cardizem vials contain 5 mg/mL. To administer the bolus you would give _____ mL over 2 minutes. To mix the continuous infusion you would inject 125 mg in a 100-mL bag of NSS. You would add _____ mL of Cardizem to the IV bag. Remembering the new total volume in the IV bag, you would set the infusion pump at _____ mL/hr to deliver 10 mg/hr.

9. Dopamine 800 mg in 250 mL D5W is infusing at 12 mL/hr in a patient weighing 195 lbs. You would document that the patient is receiving _____ mcg/kg/min.

> ### Critical Thinking Check:
>
> If the flow rate were to increase to 18 mL/hr, would you expect the mcg/kg/min to _____
> **Increase or Decrease?**

10. The physician prescribes Neo-synephrine 100 mg in 250 mL D5W continuous infusion to run at 50 mcg/min. You would set the infusion pump at _____ mL/hr. To maintain the systolic BP above 90 mmHg, the rate is increased to 12 mL/hr. You document that the patient is now receiving _____ mcg/min.

11. Aggrastat 12.5 mg in 250 mL is prescribed to be infused at a rate of 0.1 mcg/kg/min in a patient weighing 82 kg. You would set the pump at _____ mL/hr.

12. A hypertensive patient weighs 165 pounds. His physician prescribed Nipride 3 mcg/kg/min, IV. Nipride 50 mg is added to a 250-mL solution of D5W. This solution would contain a concentration of Nipride, _____ mcg/mL. Using an infusion pump, the nurse would set the flow rate at _____ mL/hr.

13. A patient is to receive Nitrostat 20 mcg/min, IV. Nitrostat is available in a 10-mL vial labeled

5 mg/mL. To prepare a 200-mcg/mL solution, with a concentration of 50 mg in 250 mL, the nurse would add _____ mL of Nitrostat to 250 mL of D5W and set the infusion pump flow rate at _____ mL/hr to deliver 20 mcg/min.

14. Give 400 mg of dopamine in 250 mL of D5NSS to infuse at 300 mcg/min. Calculate flow rate in mL/hr. You would give _____ mL/hr.

✔ **Critical Thinking Check:**

If the infusion increased to 500 mcg/min, would you expect the mL/hr to _____ **Increase or Decrease?** If the quantity of solution increased to 500 mL of D5NSS, at the same infusion of 300 mcg/min, would the mL/hr _____ **Increase or Decrease?**

---

15. A patient is started on a Lasix infusion to promote diuresis. Lasix 2,000 mg in 200 mL is prescribed at 1 mg/min. You would set the pump at _____ mL/hr.

16. A patient is started on norepinephrine 4 mg in 250 mL D5W at 15 mL/hr. You document that the patient is receiving _____ mcg/min.

17. Sandostatin 1,250 mcg in 250 mL is prescribed at 50 mcg/hr. Using an infusion pump, you would set the rate at _____ mL/hr.

18. A patient is to receive dobutamine 1,000 mg in 250 mL NSS at 10 mcg/kg/min to maintain a systolic BP of 90 mm Hg. In a patient weighing 95 kg, you would set the pump at _____ mL/hr.

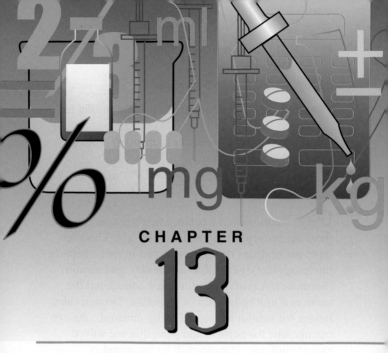

Insulin

LEARNING OBJECTIVES

After completing this chapter, you should be able to:

- Explain the purpose of insulin.
- List the different types of insulin.
- Compare the four different insulin types (rapid acting, short acting, intermediate acting and long acting) according to onset, peak and duration.
- Distinguish between three types of insulin syringes: a standard U-100 syringe, a Lo-Dose U-50 syringe and a Lo-Dose U-30 syringe.

Drugs are measured in units when strength can be more accurately determined than weight. There are three major drugs that are measured in units: heparin (anticoagulant), penicillin (antibiotic), and insulin (hormone). A unit of insulin is not considered the same as a unit of heparin or penicillin. Dosage calculations for insulin are solved using units/mL; dosage calculations for heparin and penicillin are solved using milliliters. Heparin will be presented in Chapter 14 and penicillin was already covered in Chapter 10. This chapter will focus on insulin.

Types of Insulin

Insulin is a natural hormone secreted by the beta cells of the pancreas in the islets of Langerhans to maintain blood sugar levels. Insulin enables the body to use glucose as a source of energy. Insulin is classified according to its onset, peak, and duration of action. Capital letters are used to identify types of insulin: R (regular), L (lente), U (ultralente), and N (NPH, neutral protein Hagedorn). These letters are found in large print on the insulin drug label. Regular and NPH are the two most commonly prescribed insulins. *Regular insulin is the only insulin that can be given IV!* It is also clear and colorless. All other insulins are cloudy

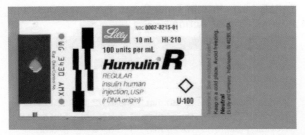

FIGURE 13.1 Humulin R (Courtesy of Eli Lilly Company, Indianapolis, Indiana).

in the vial. Never shake the insulin vial! Always mix by rolling between the palms of your hands.

See Figures 13.1 and 13.2 for two common types of insulin. See Table 13.1 for a breakdown of insulin type and action.

Insulin Preparations

Insulin is measured in units and is most commonly supplied in 10-mL vials providing 100 units of insulin/mL (U = 100/mL). The standard U-100 insulin syringe is used. Insulin comes in fixed, combination preparations. The ratio of the combined insulin always equals 100% (Humalog Mix 50/50). Therefore, if a physician orders

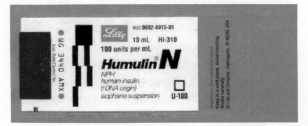

FIGURE 13.2 Humulin N (Courtesy of Eli Lilly Company, Indianapolis, Indiana).

TABLE 13.1 Insulin Type, Onset, Peak, and Duration of Action

INSULIN	ONSET	PEAK	DURATION
Rapid Acting			
Aprida (glulisine)	15–30 min	1/2–2 1/2 hr	5 hr or less
Humalog (lispro)	15–30 min	1/2–2 1/2 hr	5 hr or less
NovoLog (aspart)	10–20 min	1–3 hr	3–5 hr
Short Acting			
Humulin R (Regular)	1/2–1 hr	2–4 hr	5–8 hr
Novolin R (Regular)	1/2 hr	2 1/2–5 hr	8 hr
ReliOn R (Novolin R)	1/2 hr	2 1/2–5 hr	8 hr
Intermediate Acting			
Humulin N (NPH)	1–2 hr	2–8 hr	14–24 hr
Novolin N (NPH)	1 1/2 hr	4–12 hr	24 hr
ReliOn N (Novolin N)	1 1/2 hr	4–12 hr	24 hr
Long Acting			
Lantus (insulin glargine)	1 1/2 hr	No	20–24 hr
Levemir (insulin detemir)	1–2 hr	No	24 hr

30 units of Humalog 50/50, you would prepare 15 U of lispro protamine and 15 U of insulin lispro.

Two insulin combination preparations are commonly available, Humulin 70/30 combination (70% NPH, 30% Regular) and a 50/50 combination (50% lispro protamine and 50% insulin lispro).

Insulin Syringes

Insulin, which is supplied in units, is given with specialized syringes, U-100s. The most common U-100 syringe is calibrated every 2 units, with every 10th unit marked in large numbers on one side (Figure 13.3A). A double-scale U-100 syringe has 2-unit calibrations. Every 5 units is marked in large numbers on the left side, and every 10 units is marked on the

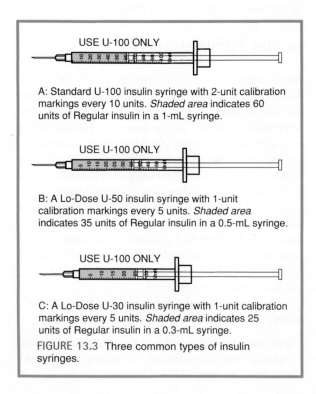

A: Standard U-100 insulin syringe with 2-unit calibration markings every 10 units. *Shaded area* indicates 60 units of Regular insulin in a 1-mL syringe.

B: A Lo-Dose U-50 insulin syringe with 1-unit calibration markings every 5 units. *Shaded area* indicates 35 units of Regular insulin in a 0.5-mL syringe.

C: A Lo-Dose U-30 insulin syringe with 1-unit calibration markings every 5 units. *Shaded area* indicates 25 units of Regular insulin in a 0.3-mL syringe.

FIGURE 13.3 Three common types of insulin syringes.

right side. This makes it easier to accurately measure odd and even unit increments.

A U-50 Lo-Dose insulin syringe is calibrated in 50 units/mL. There are 1-unit calibration markings every 5 units. The U-50 syringe holds 0.5 mL. A U-30 syringe also has 1-unit calibrations every 5 units (Figure 13.3 B & C). The U-30 syringe holds 0.3 mL. The enlarged scale of the Lo-Dose syringe makes it easier to read. Insulin is also available in prefilled, disposable pens or cartridges for reusable pens. Continuous insulin infusion pumps deliver a set dose of rapid-acting insulin on an hourly basis.

Insulin Administration

Insulin orders are written in units/mL and U-100 strength is used almost exclusively. Orders must include the type of insulin (Regular, Humulin N), the units, the route (subcutaneous), and the time (e.g., 1/2 hour before meals, at bedtime). Some patients receive additional insulin during the day to "cover" for excess blood sugar. A sliding scale (blood sugar of 300 mg/dL = 6 U of Regular) is used with regular or lispro insulin.

With U-100 medication orders, all you have to do is draw up the desired dose by filling the insulin syringe to the identified calibration. Remember: Only prepare insulin in an insulin syringe and only use a U-100 syringe for U-100 insulin. Mathematical calculations will not be required.

To prepare insulin for injection, follow these steps:

• Read the medication order, noting the type of insulin and unit preparation desired. For example, a patient is ordered 60 units of NPH insulin.

- Select the insulin vial. Check the vial label three times. You should choose the vial of NPH insulin marked 100 units/mL.
- Match the insulin syringe to the unit preparation of insulin. You should choose a U-100 syringe because the insulin preparation comes in a vial marked 100 U/mL.
- Draw up the required dose by filling the syringe to the desired calibration. You would fill a U-100 syringe to the 60 units calibration.

Mixing Two Types of Insulin

Frequently you will find it necessary to mix two types of insulin, usually Regular and NPH. Lantus should never be mixed in a syringe with another insulin. When you have to mix insulins, there are *five important guidelines that you must remember:*

1. Do not contaminate the contents of one vial with the contents of the other vial.
2. Always draw up *Regular insulin first.*
3. Always *draw up the NPH insulin last* because chemically it has a protein substance in it that Regular insulin does not have. Drawing up the NPH insulin last helps prevent contamination of the Regular insulin.
4. Choose a Lo-Dose insulin syringe (U-30 or U-50) to measure low dosages; use a U-100 syringe for insulin combinations.
5. Always add air into each vial equal to the amount of the required dose. Air prevents a vacuum from occurring. *Note:* Always inject air into the *NPH vial first!*

To mix two types of insulin in one syringe for injection, Regular and NPH, follow these steps and refer to the illustrations A–G.

- Check the medication order. Know the total number of units needed.
- Wash your hands and obtain the correct vials of insulin and the correct syringes. Both should be in the same unit of strength (U-100).
- Wipe the top of both vials with an alcohol swab. Regular is always clear and colorless in appearance. NPH is cloudy in appearance. Rotate the vial of NPH between your palms. *Never shake the vial.*
- Inject air equal to the insulin dose of NPH (20 units) into the NPH insulin vial first (**A**). *Do not touch the insulin solution with the tip of the needle.* Withdraw the needle.

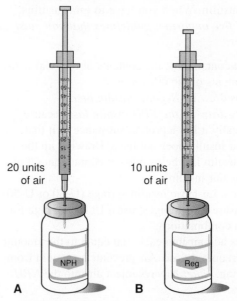

20 units of air

10 units of air

A   **B**

- Use the same syringe and inject air equal to the dose of Regular insulin (10 units) into the Regular insulin vial (**B**). Be careful that the needle does not touch the solution because air should not be bubbled through the solution.
- Invert the vial of Regular insulin and draw back the required dosage (**C**). Check the dosage (10 units).
- Remove the needle from the vial of Regular insulin (**D**) and check for air bubbles. Tap the syringe to remove any bubbles. If necessary, draw up additional medication for correct dosage.

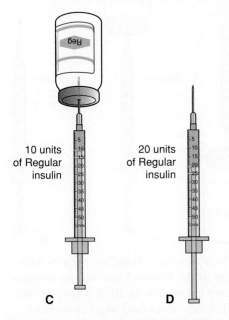

10 units of Regular insulin

20 units of Regular insulin

C

D

- Put the needle into the NPH vial (**E**), being careful not to inject any Regular insulin into the NPH vial.
- Invert the vial of NPH and withdraw the required dosage (20 units) while holding the syringe

at eye level. There should be a total of 30 units (**F**).

- Check the dosage, which should be the addition of the two insulin orders (**G**). Air bubbles at this point indicate an incorrect dose, and the medication must be drawn up again.
- Prepare to administer the correct dose.

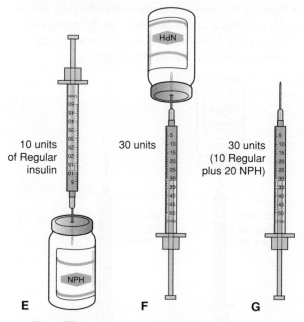

10 units
of Regular
insulin

30 units

30 units
(10 Regular
plus 20 NPH)

E   F   G

Note: There are over 180 million persons with diabetes in the world. Research into insulin management is progressing rapidly. In 2007, a new, needle-free device that measures blood sugar using near-infrared rays was successfully piloted in China and experimental islet cell transplants took place in the United States.

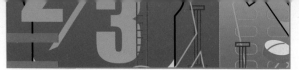

End of Chapter Review

Look at the following syringes and identify the correct dosage of insulin by using an arrow to mark your answer or shade in the areas.

1. Indicate 60 units U-100 insulin.

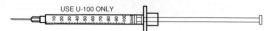

2. Indicate 82 units U-100 insulin.

USE U-100 ONLY

3. Indicate 45 units U-100 insulin.

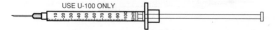

4. Indicate 35 units U-100 insulin.

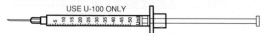

5. Indicate 10 units Regular U-100 insulin combined with 16 units NPH U-100 insulin.

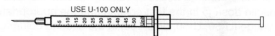

6. Indicate 16 units Regular U-100 insulin combined with 40 units NPH U-100 insulin.

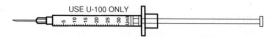

Identify the insulin dosage indicated by the shaded area on the following syringes.

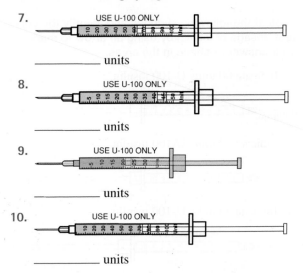

7. USE U-100 ONLY

_____ units

8. USE U-100 ONLY

_____ units

9. USE U-100 ONLY

_____ units

10. USE U-100 ONLY

_____ units

For the combined doses of insulin, indicate the total insulin dosage in the first column and the appropriate syringe (U-30, U-50, or U-100) in the second column.

	Total Dosage	Syringe/mL
11. 5 U Regular 16 U NPH	_____	_____
12. 30 NPH 15 U Regular	_____	_____
13. 28 U Regular 36 U NPH	_____	_____
14. 18 U Regular 20 U NPH	_____	_____
15. 20 NPH 10 U Regular	_____	_____

16. The physician ordered 30 U of U-100 Regular insulin to be given before lunch. You would select a _____ syringe and draw up _____ U of Regular insulin.

Critical Thinking Check:

Does it seem logical or not logical to use a U-100 syringe because the Regular insulin is U-100? _____ **Logical or Not Logical?**

---

17. You have been asked to give 15 U of Humulin R insulin and 24 U of U-100 NPH. You would give a combined dose of _____ units in a _____ syringe.

18. The physician prescribed 15 units of Humulin R insulin to be given subcutaneously at 11:00 AM to cover an "Accucheck" reading of 325. The nurse would use a U-30 syringe and draw up _____ units.

19. The physician prescribed 50 units of Humulin N insulin to be given subcutaneously at 8:00 AM. Using a U-100 insulin syringe, the nurse would draw up _____ units.

Critical Thinking Check:

Does it seem logical or not logical to use a U-100 syringe for 50 units of Humulin N? _____ **Logical or Not Logical?**

20. The physician prescribed a combination of 22 units of NPH insulin and 12 units of Regular insulin. Using a U-100 insulin syringe, the nurse would draw up a total of _____ units, making certain to draw up the _____ insulin last.

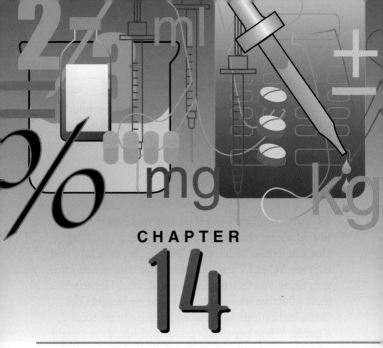

Heparin Preparation and Dosage Calculations

LEARNING OBJECTIVES

After completing this chapter, you should be able to:

- Explain the purpose of heparin.
- Calculate heparin for subcutaneous injection.
- Calculate heparin for intravenous infusion.

- Calculate heparin flow rate in milliliters per hour.
- Calculate heparin flow rate in units per hour.
- Calculate heparin flow rate using weight-based heparin.

Heparin is an anticoagulant that prevents the formation of a new clot and the extension of an existing clot. Heparin is ordered in U/hr, mg/hr, or mL/hr and is given SC or IV for intermittent or continuous infusion using an electronic infusion device. Heparin is most effective when ordered based on weight (kg). Some institutions will use an IV heparin protocol as a guide. When heparin is prescribed based on weight, a bolus is ordered in units/kg, followed by a continuous heparin infusion prescribed in U/kg/hr and given via an electronic infusion device.

To safely administer heparin, first read the vial label carefully! There are several different dosage strengths from Heparin Lock Flush (10 U/mL) to Heparin Solution (10,000 U/mL). Next, determine that the prescribed dose is within normal limits and can safely be given based on the patient's coagulation laboratory test results, the activated partial thromboplastin time (PTT). Then, verify the route of administration and calculate the 24-hour dosage to estimate safety of drug administration.

Heparin comes in various solution strengths of units/mL: 10, 100, 1,000, 10,000, 20,000, and 40,000. Subcutaneous heparin works in 20 to 60 minutes, whereas IV heparin is immediate. The normal

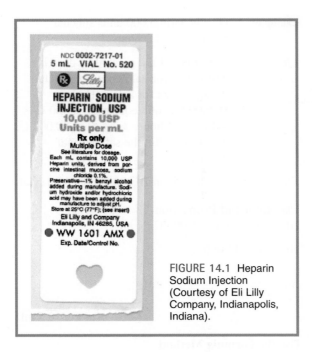

NDC 0002-7217-01
5 mL   VIAL No. 520

Ⓡ *Lilly*

**HEPARIN SODIUM
INJECTION, USP**
10,000 USP
Units per mL
Rx only
Multiple Dose
See literature for dosage.
Each mL contains 10,000 USP
Heparin units, derived from por-
cine intestinal mucosa, sodium
chloride 0.1%.
Preservative—1% benzyl alcohol
added during manufacture. Sodi-
um hydroxide and/or hydrochloric
acid may have been added during
manufacture to adjust pH.
Store at 25°C (77°F); (see insert)
Eli Lilly and Company
Indianapolis, IN 46285, USA
● WW 1601 AMX ●
Exp. Date/Control No.

FIGURE 14.1 Heparin
Sodium Injection
(Courtesy of Eli Lilly
Company, Indianapolis,
Indiana).

heparinizing adult dosage is 20,000 U to 40,000
U/24 hours. See Figure 14.1.

Calculate Heparin for Subcutaneous Injection

RULE: To prepare heparin for subcutaneous injection, you
would: determine that the dosage is within the normal
range and use one of three methods to calculate dosages;
use a tuberculin or prepackaged syringe to administer.

Example: Give heparin 5,000 units subcutaneously every 6 hours.

Check: Determine if the prescribed dose is within the normal heparinizing adult dosage range for safety. Heparin @ 5,000 U, q6h equates to 5,000 U × 4 doses (24 hours ÷ by 6) = 20,000 U, which is within the safe normal dosage.

Select: Select heparin 10,000 U/mL; 5-mL vial

Use Ratio and Proportion

10,000 U : 1 mL :: 5,000 U : x mL

$10,000x = 15,000$

$x = \dfrac{15,000}{10,000} = \dfrac{5}{10} = 0.5$ mL

Answer: 0.5 mL

Use the Formula Method

$\dfrac{D}{H} \times Q = x$

$\dfrac{5,000 \text{ U}}{10,000 \text{ U}} = \dfrac{1}{2}$

$\dfrac{1}{2} \times 1.0$ mL $= 0.5$ mL

Answer: 0.5 mL

Use Dimensional Analysis

x mL $= \dfrac{1 \text{ mL}}{10,000} \times \dfrac{5,000 \text{ U}}{1}$

$$x \, \text{mL} = \frac{5,000}{10,000} = \frac{5}{10} = 0.5$$

Answer: 0.5 mL

Example: A patient is prescribed 3,000 units of heparin to be administered subcutaneously every 12 hours.

Check: Determine if the prescribed dose is within the normal heparinizing adult dosage for 24 hours. Heparin @ 3,000 U, q12h = 6,000 U/24 hours. This is below the normal dosage range and is safe to give.

Select: Select the appropriate ampule/vial. For example, you would choose a 10-mL multidose vial in a concentration of 5,000 units/mL.

Use Ratio and Proportion

5,000 U : 1 mL :: 3,000 U : x mL

$5,000x = 3,000$

$$x = \frac{3,000}{5,000} = \frac{3}{5} = 0.6 \, \text{mL}$$

Answer: 0.6 mL

Use the Formula Method

$$\frac{D}{H} \times Q = x$$

$$\frac{3,000 \, \text{U}}{5,000 \, \text{U}} = \frac{3}{5}$$

$\dfrac{3}{5} \times 1.0$ mL (quantity) $= 0.6$ mL

Answer: 0.6 mL

Use Dimensional Analysis

x mL $= \dfrac{1 \text{ mL}}{5,000 \text{ U}} \times \dfrac{3,000 \text{ U}}{1}$

x mL $= \dfrac{3,000}{5,000} = \dfrac{3}{5} = 0.6$ mL

Answer: 0.6 mL

Calculate Heparin for Intravenous Infusion

Heparin Flow Rate: Calculate Hourly Dosage

When the physician orders the flow rate for an infusion of heparin, you must calculate the hourly dose to verify that the 24-hour dosage is within a safe range.

> **RULE: To calculate the hourly dosage of heparin for intravenous infusion when the flow rate is prescribed, you would: use either ratio and proportion or Dimensional Analysis to calculate the hourly units of heparin and then verify that the dosage is within the normal heparinizing adult range.**

| Example: | Give 1,000 mL of D5W with 30,000 units of heparin to infuse at 50 mL/hr. |

Use Ratio and Proportion

30,000 U : 1,000 mL :: x U : 50 mL

$1,000 \times x = 30,000 \times 50$

$1,000x = 1,500,000$

Solve for x: $x = \dfrac{1,500,000}{1,000} = 1,500$ U/hr

$x = 1,500$ U in 50 mL to infuse per hour

Answer: 1,500 U/hr

Use Dimensional Analysis

x U/hr $= \dfrac{30,000 \text{ U/hr}}{1,000 \text{ mL}} \times \dfrac{50 \text{ mL}}{1 \text{ hr}}$

x U/hr $= \dfrac{30,000}{1,000} \times \dfrac{50}{1} = \dfrac{30}{1} \times \dfrac{50}{1} = 1,500$

Answer: 1,500 U/hr

| *Estimate 24-Hour Dosage:* | 1,500 U/hr $\times$ 24 hr = 36,000 U/24 hr. This is within the normal adult range. |

RULE: To calculate the hourly dosage of heparin for intravenous infusion when the calibration (gtt/mL) and flow rate (gtt/min) are known, you would: convert gtt/min to mL/min, change mL/min to mL/hr, and then use ratio and proportion or Dimensional Analysis to calculate units/hr.

Example: Give 1,000 mL D5W with 20,000 U of heparin by straight gravity flow infusion. The drop factor is 10 gtt/mL, and the IV flow rate is 10 gtt/min. Calculate the hourly dosage of heparin.

Calculate mL/min:
10 gtt : 1 mL :: 10 gtt : x mL/min

$10x = 10$

$x = 1$ mL/min

Change mL/min to mL/hr:
1 mL/min $\times$ 60 min = 60 mL/hr

Use Ratio and Proportion

20,000 U : 1,000 mL :: x U : 60 mL

$1,000 \times x = 20,000 \times 60$

$1,000x = 1,200,000$

$\dfrac{1,000\,x}{1,000} = \dfrac{1,200,000}{1,000}$

$x = \dfrac{\cancel{1,200,000}^{\,1200}}{\cancel{1,000}_{\,1}}$

$x = 1,200$ U/hr

Answer: 1,200 U/hr

Use Dimensional Analysis

x U/hr $= \dfrac{20,000 \text{ U}}{1,000 \text{ mL}} \times \dfrac{60 \text{ mL}}{1}$

x U/hr $= \dfrac{20}{1} \times 60 = 1,200$ U/hr

Answer: 1,200 U/hr

Estimate	1,200 U × 24 hr = 28,800/24 hr. This
24-Hour	is within the normal range for adult
Dosage:	dosage.

Heparin Flow Rate: Calculate Milliliters per Hour

RULE: To calculate flow rate (mL/hr) when heparin is ordered in units per hour you would: use either ratio and proportion or Dimensional Analysis to solve for *x*. Calculate the flow rate in gtt/min if the infusion is by gravity. Use the Quick Formula with a constant factor, if possible.

Example: Give 1,000 U/hr of heparin IV. You have 500 mL of D5W with 20,000 U of heparin added. The drop factor is 15 gtt/mL. Calculate the flow rate.

Use Ratio and Proportion

20,000 U : 500 mL :: 1,000 U : x mL

$20,000x = 500 \times 1,000$

$20,000x = 500,000$

$\dfrac{20,000\,x}{20,000} = \dfrac{500,000}{20,000}$

$x = \dfrac{\cancel{20,000}^{\uparrow x}}{\cancel{20,000}_{\uparrow}} = \dfrac{\cancel{500,000}^{25}}{\cancel{20,000}_{\uparrow}}$

$x = 25$ mL/hr

Answer: 25 mL/hr

Use Dimensional Analysis

$$x \text{ mL/hr} = \frac{500 \text{ mL}}{20,000 \text{ U}} \times \frac{1,000 \text{ U}}{1}$$

$$x \text{ mL/hr} = \frac{500}{20} \times 1 = \frac{50}{2} = 25 \times 1 = 25 \text{ mL/hr}$$

Answer: 25 mL/hr

Calculate gtt/min— Use:

$$\frac{\text{mL/hr}}{\text{constant factor}} = \text{gtt/min}$$

$$\frac{25 \text{ mL/hr}}{4} = 6.25 \text{ gtt/min}$$

Round off to 6 gtt/min

Answer: 6 gtt/min

Example: Give 600 U/hr of heparin IV. You have 1,000 mL of D5W with 25,000 U of heparin added. The drop factor is 60 gtt/min (microdrops). Calculate the flow rate.

Use Ratio and Proportion

25,000 U : 1,000 mL :: 600 U : x mL

$$25,000x = 1,000 \times 600$$

$$25,000x = 600,000$$

$$\frac{25,000 \, x}{25,000} = \frac{600,000}{25,000}$$

$$\frac{\cancel{25,000}^{1} x}{\cancel{25,000}_{1}} = \frac{\cancel{600,000}^{24}}{\cancel{25,000}_{1}}$$

$$x = 24 \text{ mL/hr}$$

Answer: 24 mL/hr

Use Dimensional Analysis

$$x \text{ mL/hr} = \frac{1,000 \text{ mL}}{25,000 \text{ U}} \times \frac{600 \text{ U}}{1}$$

$$x \text{ mL/hr} = \frac{1}{25} \times 600 = 24 \text{ mL/hr}$$

Answer: 24 mL/hr

Calculate gtt/min— Use:

$$\frac{\text{mL/hr}}{\text{constant factor}} = \text{gtt/min}$$

$$\frac{24 \text{ mL/hr}}{1} = 24 \text{ gtt/min}$$

Answer: 24 gtt/min

Heparin Flow Rate: Calculate Units per Hour

> **RULE: To calculate units per hour when heparin is ordered in mL/hr, you would: use ratio and proportion or Dimensional Analysis to solve for *x*. Estimate safe dosage range.**

Example: Give 1,000 mL of D5W with 30,000 units of heparin to infuse at 30 mL/hr. Calculate the hourly dosage of heparin.

Use Ratio and Proportion

30,000 U : 1,000 mL :: *x* U : 30 mL

1,000 × *x* = 30,000 × 30

1,000*x* = 900,000

$$x = \frac{\cancel{900,000}}{\cancel{1,000}_1} = 900$$

$$x = 900 \text{ U/hr}$$

Answer: 900 U/hr

Use Dimensional Analysis

$$x \text{ U/hr} = \frac{30,000 \text{ U}}{1,000 \text{ mL}} \times \frac{30 \text{ mL}}{1}$$

$$x \text{ U/hr} = \frac{30,000}{1,000} \times \frac{30}{1} = \frac{30}{1} \times 30 = 900 \text{ U/hr}$$

Answer: 900 U/hr

Estimate   900 U/hr × 24 hr = 21,600 U/24 hr.
24-Hour   This is within the normal range for
Dosage: adult dosage (20,000–40,000 U/24 hr).

Heparin Flow Rate: Calculating Weight-Based Heparin

> **RULE: To calculate the flow rate (mL/hr) when the units/kg/hr are known, you would: convert to like units (lbs to kg), calculate units/hr, and calculate mL/hr using one of the three methods to calculate dosages. The Formula Method will be used here.**

Example: A physician orders heparin 12,500 units in 250 mL D5W to run at 16 units/kg/hr in a patient weighing 124 pounds. The nurse should set the infusion pump at _____ mL/hr.

Convert
lbs to kg

124 lbs ÷ 2.2 lbs/kg = 56.4 kg
Round to the nearest tenth (56 kg)

Calculate
units/hr:

16 units/kg/hr × 56 kg
= 896 units/hr

Calculate
mL/hr
Using the
Formula
Method:

$$\frac{D}{H} \times Q = mL/hr$$

Solve for x:

$$\frac{896 \text{ units/hr}}{12{,}500 \text{ units}} \times 250 \text{ mL}$$

= 17.75 or 18 mL/hr

Answer: Set the infusion pump
at 18 mL/hr

> RULE: To calculate units/kg/hr when the flow rate (mL/hr)
> is known, you would: convert to like units (lbs to kg) and
> calculate the units/hr using one of three methods. The
> Formula Method will be used here.

Example:

Heparin 12,500 units in 250 mL D5W
is infusing at 15 mL/hr in a patient
weighing 189 pounds. How many
units/kg/hr is the patient receiving?

Convert
lbs to kg

189 lbs ÷ 2.2 lbs/kg = 86 kg

Calculate
units/hr
Using the
Formula
Method:

$$\frac{x \text{ units/hr}}{12{,}500 \text{ units}} \times 250 \text{ mL} = 15 \text{ mL/hr}$$

Solve for x: $12{,}500 \times \dfrac{x \text{ units/hr}}{12{,}500 \text{ units}} \times 250 \text{ mL}$

$= 15 \text{ mL/hr} \times 12{,}500$

$x \times 250 \text{ mL} \div 250 \text{ mL} = 187{,}500 \div 250$

$x = 750 \text{ units/hr}$

Calculate units/kg/hr: $750 \text{ units/hr} \div 86 \text{ kg} = 8.7 \text{ units/kg/hr}$

Answer: 8.7 units/kg/hr

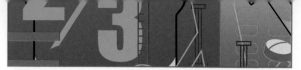

End of Chapter Review

1. Give 500 mL of D5 NSS with 10,000 units of heparin to infuse at 20 mL/hr. Calculate the hourly dosage of heparin. Is the dosage within the normal, safe range for 24 hours?

   Answer = _____ U/hr. Safe or unsafe? _____

2. Give 1,000 mL of D5W with 20,000 U of heparin IV. The drop factor is 20 gtt/mL, and the IV flow rate is 10 gtt/min. Calculate the hourly dosage of heparin. Is the dosage within the normal, safe range for 24 hours? _____

   Answer = _____ U/hr. Safe or unsafe? _____

3. Give 800 U of heparin IV every hour. You have 1,000 mL of D5 NSS with 40,000 U of heparin added. The drop factor is 60 gtt/min. Calculate the flow rate.

   Answer = _____ mL/hr _____ gtt/min

4. The physician prescribes a heparin bolus of 80 units/kg followed by an infusion of heparin 12,500 units in 250 mL D5W to run at 18 units/kg/hr in a patient weighing 56 kg. You should administer _____ units IV push for the bolus and start the infusion at _____ mL/hr.

5. The results of a PTT blood test came back for the above patient and the protocol directs you to increase the infusion by 2 units/kg/hr. After recalculating the rate you set the infusion pump at _____ mL/hr.

Critical Thinking Check:

Since the infusion was increased, can you assume that the patient's PTT result was equal to, greater than, or less than the previous reading and the control? _____ **Equal to, Less Than, or Greater Than?**

6. Heparin 12,500 units in 250 mL D5W is infusing at 21 mL/hr in a patient who weighs 92 kg. How many U/kg/hr is the patient receiving at this flow rate? _____

7. A patient is to receive 10,000 units of heparin subcutaneously at 8:00 AM and 8:00 PM for 5 days. Heparin sodium for injection is available in a TUBEX Cartridge-Needle unit in 15,000 units/mL. The nurse would give _____ mL every 12 hours for a daily total dosage of _____ U/24 hours. This is/is not within the normal dosage range. _____

8. Heparin sodium, 8,000 units, is to be given subcutaneously, every 8 hours. The medication is available in a vial labeled 10,000 units per milliliter. The nurse would give _____ mL every 8 hours for a total dosage of _____ U/24 hr. This is/is not within the normal dosage range. _____

Critical Thinking Check:

If an alternate dosage was prescribed for this patient, which daily dosage would you recognize as unsafe to give: _____ **10,000 U/8 hr; 12,000 U/8 hr; or 15,000 U/8 hr?**

9. The physician prescribed heparin sodium, 5,000 units, subcutaneously, twice a day. Heparin is available in a vial labeled 7,500 units per milliliter. The nurse would give _____ mL twice a day for a total dosage of _____ U/24 hr. This is/is not within the normal dosage range. _____

10. The physician prescribed 5,000 units of heparin for injection intravenously through a heparin lock. Heparin is available in a 10-mL vial in a concentration of 20,000 units per milliliter. The nurse would administer _____ mL.

11. The physician ordered 500 mL of D5W with 30,000 units of heparin to infuse at 10 mL/hr. Calculate the hourly dosage of heparin: _____ U/hr in 10 mL.

12. The physician prescribed 1,000 mL of 0.45% NSS with 15,000 U of heparin IV. The drop factor is 10 gtt/mL, and the IV flow rate is 15 gtt/min. Calculate the hourly dosage of heparin: _____ mL/ min = _____ mL/hr; give _____ U/hr = _____ U/24 hr.

13. You are to give 500 U of heparin IV hourly. You have 1,000 mL D5W with 10,000 U of heparin added. The drop factor is 20 gtt/mL. Calculate the flow rate: _____ mL/hr will be infused at _____ gtt/min.

14. A patient is to receive 500 mL of D5W with 15,000 units of heparin over 24 hours. The drop factor is 60 gtt/mL. Using an infusion pump, the nurse would set the flow rate at _____ mL/hr to deliver _____ units/hr of heparin.

15. Give 500 units/hr of heparin IV. You have 500 mL of D5W with 10,000 units of heparin added. The drop factor is 15 gtt/mL. Calculate the flow rate. _____

16. The activated PTT is elevated and the protocol directs you to hold the heparin (12,500 units in 250 mL D5W) infusion for 1 hour and restart it at 10 units/kg/hr. If the patient weighs 140 pounds, how many mL/hr should the patient receive? _____

17. Heparin 12,500 units in 250 mL D5W is infusing at 15 mL/hr in a patient weighing 126 pounds. You would document that the patient is receiving _____ units/kg/hr.

CHAPTER 15

Pediatric Dosage Calculations and Intravenous Therapy

LEARNING OBJECTIVES

After completing this chapter, you should be able to:

- Explain the concept of body surface area (BSA) using the West nomogram.
- Convert weight in pounds to kilograms.
- Convert weight in kilograms to pounds.

- Determine safe dosage range for calculated amounts.
- Calculate oral and parenteral dosages.
- Calculate dosages using Fried's Rule, Young's Rule, and Clark's Rule.
- Calculate dosages using body surface area and a nomogram.

Extreme care must be taken when preparing and administering medications to infants (birth to 12 months) and children (age 1–12 years). Dosages are estimated based on age, size, weight, height, body surface area, and physical condition. Dosages are calculated using either body weight (mg/kg) or body surface area (BSA) using the West nomogram. You need to become comfortable calculating pediatric medications using dosages per kilogram of body weight (1 kg = 2.2 lbs) and dosages determined by Fried's Rule, Clark's Rule, and Young's Rule. Whenever calculating dosages, *always compare the prescribed dosage to the recommended dosage using a reference drug resource* to determine the safe dosage.

Oral pediatric medications are prescribed in liquid form whenever possible. Because dosages are so small and exact, you need to review and be comfortable with calculations using micrograms (1,000 mg = 1 mcg). *Parenteral* medications are most commonly given via the subcutaneous and intramuscular routes. Dosage amount is limited to 1 mL per site for those under 5 years of age (usually 0.5 mL for infants) and the quantity is measured using a tuberculin syringe. Refer to Appendix E for information on subcutaneous injections and Appendix H for pediatric intramuscular injections. Appendix I covers Nursing Concerns for Pediatric Drug Administration.

It is essential that pediatric *intravenous* therapy be as exact as possible because infants and children have a narrow range of fluid balance. Therefore, a volume-controlled infusion set is recommended, and total fluid volume consists of medication diluent volume, IV solution volume, and flush volume (5–15 mL). An intravenous infusion rate is calculated in both gtt/min and mL/hr using a microdrip (60 gtt/min) or electronic device.

Converting Weight in Pounds to Kilograms

Sometimes medications are prescribed in milligrams/kilogram of body weight. Because there are 2.2 pounds in 1 kilogram, you must convert the child's weight in pounds to kilograms before you can calculate the drug dosage. The following rule tells you how to calculate drug dosages when the drug is ordered according to kilograms of body weight.

> **RULE: To convert pounds to kilograms, you would:** *divide* the patient's body weight in pounds by 2.2. To convert kilograms to pounds, you would: *multiply* the patient's body weight in kilograms by 2.2. *Note:* for premature infants, you will probably need to work with grams (1,000 grams = 1 kilogram).

Example:

Convert 44 lbs to kg: Move the decimal point in the divisor and the dividend the same number of places. Put the decimal point directly above the line for the quotient.

$$2.2. \overline{)44.0.}$$

$$\frac{20.}{22)440.} \text{ (quotient)}$$

Answer: 20 kg

Calculate Oral and Parenteral Dosages

> **RULE: To calculate a pediatric oral or parenteral medication dosage, you would: convert pounds to kilograms, solve for x, and estimate the safe dosage range and the total 24-hour amount.**

Example: The physician prescribed amoxicillin 20 mg/kg/day to be administered q8h in equally divided doses. The patient weighed 44 pounds (20 kg) and was 5 years old. The safe dosage range for amoxicillin is 20 to 40 mg/kg/day.

Use Ratio and Proportion

20 mg : 1 kg :: x mg : 20 kg

$1x = 20 \times 20$

$1x = 400$

$x = 400$ mg

Estimate   400 mg will be divided into three equal
Dosage: doses. 400 mg ÷ 3 = 133 mg to be
                given every 8 hours.

Answer: 133 mg/dose

Use Dimensional Analysis

$$x \text{ mg} = \frac{20 \text{ mg}}{1 \text{ kg}} \times \frac{20 \text{ kg}}{1}$$

$$x = \frac{20}{1} \times \frac{20}{1} = 400 \text{ mg} \div 3 = 133 \text{ mg to be given}$$
every 8 hours

Answer: 133 mg/dose

Estimate Safe Dosage Range Using Either Ratio and Proportion or Dimensional Analysis

After you calculate the amount of medication to give, compare that amount with the total recommended safe dosage. *Note:* drug labels indicate the recommended daily (24-hour) safe dosage range in mg/kg.

Use Ratio and Proportion

The safe dosage range for amoxicillin is 20–40 mg/ kg/day.

20 mg : 1 kg :: x mg : 20 kg

$1x = 20 \times 20 = 400$ mg/day

40 mg : 1 kg :: x mg : 20 kg

$1x = 40 \times 20 = 800$ mg/day

Answer: 400–800 mg/day

Use Dimensional Analysis

$$x = \frac{20 \text{ mg}}{1 \text{ kg}} \times \frac{20 \text{ kg}}{1}$$

$$x = 20 \times 20 = 400 \text{ mg/day}$$

$$x = \frac{40 \text{ mg}}{1 \text{ kg}} \times \frac{20 \text{ kg}}{1}$$

$$x = 40 \times 20 = 800 \text{ mg/day}$$

Answer: 400–800 mg/day

Therefore, giving 133 mg/dose × 3 doses = 400 mg/day, which is within the safe range of 400 to 800 mg/day.

Example:	The physician prescribed amoxicillin 125 mg, PO, q8h for a 33-pound child. Amoxicillin is available as 250 mg/ 5 mL. The safe dosage range is 20 to 40 mg/kg/day.
Convert:	33 pounds to kilograms
Use:	1 kg : 2.2 lbs :: x kg : 33 lbs
	$2.2x = 33$
	$x = 33 \div 2.2 = 15$ kg

Use Ratio and Proportion

125 mg : x mL :: 250 mg : 5 mL

$$250x = 5 \times 125 = 625$$

$$250x = 625$$

$$x = 2.5 \text{ mL}$$

Answer: 2.5 mL/8 hr

Use the Formula Method

Calculate: Use $\dfrac{D}{H} \times Q = x$

$$\frac{125 \text{ mg}}{250 \text{ mg}} \times 5 \text{ mL}$$

$$\frac{1}{2} \times 5 = \frac{5}{2} = 2.5 \text{ mL}$$

Answer: 2.5 mL/8 hr

Use Dimensional Analysis

$$x \text{ mL} = \frac{5 \text{ mL}}{250 \text{ mg}} \times \frac{125 \text{ mg}}{1}$$

$$x \text{ mL} = \frac{625}{250} = \frac{5}{2} = 2.5 \text{ mL}$$

Answer: 2.5 mL/8 hr

Estimate Safe Dosage Range Using Either Ratio and Proportion or Dimensional Analysis

Use Ratio and Proportion

- 20 mg : 1 kg :: x mg : 15 kg

  $1x = 15 \times 20$

  $1x = 300$ mg/day

- 40 mg : 1 kg :: x mg : 15 kg

  $1x = 40 \times 15$

  $1x = 600$ mg/day

Answer: 300–600 mg/day
is the safe dosage range

Use Dimensional Analysis

$$x = \frac{20 \text{ mg}}{1 \text{ kg}} \times \frac{15 \text{ kg}}{1}$$

$$x = 20 \times 15 = 300 \text{ mg/day}$$

$$x = \frac{40 \text{ mg}}{1 \text{ kg}} \times \frac{15 \text{ kg}}{1}$$

$$x = 40 \times 15 = 600 \text{ mg/day}$$

Answer: 300–600 mg/day

Total Amount in 24 Hours	The physician prescribed 125 mg, PO, q8h. Three doses of 125 mg = 375 mg/day. This amount (375 mg in 24 hours) falls within the safe range of 300 to 600 mg/day. (20–40 mg/kg/day)

Calculate Dosages Using Rule Based on Age

> **FRIED'S RULE: To determine dosage for newborns to 2-year-olds you would: divide the child's age in months by 150 and multiply by the adult dose. Use ratio and proportion, the Formula Method, or Dimensional Analysis to determine the amount to give.**

Example: The physician prescribed Benadryl elixir for a 15-month-old. The normal adult dose is 25 mg every 4 to 6 hours. Benadryl elixir is available as 12.5 mg/ 5 mL.

Use Fried's Rule:

$$\text{Pediatric dose} = \frac{\text{age in months}}{150}$$

$\times$ normal adult dose

$$\text{Pediatric dose} = \frac{15 \text{ months}}{150} = \frac{1}{10}$$

$\times$ 25 mg = 2.5 mg

Because Benadryl is available as 12.5 mg/5 mL, additional computation is necessary to determine the amount of milliliters to give.

Use Ratio and Proportion

2.5 mg : x :: 12.5 mg : 5 mL

$12.5x = 12.5$

$x = 1$ mL

Answer: 1 mL

Use the Formula Method

$$\frac{\text{D}}{\text{H}} \times \text{Q} = x$$

= amount to give

$$\frac{2.5 \text{ mg}}{12.5 \text{ mg}} \times 5 = \frac{1}{5} \times 5 = 1 \text{ mL}$$

Answer: 1 mL

Use Dimensional Analysis

$$x \text{ mL} = \frac{5 \text{ mL}}{12.5 \text{ mg}} \times \frac{2.5 \text{ mg}}{1}$$

$$x = \frac{12.5}{12.5} = 1 \text{ mL}$$

Answer: 1 mL

> YOUNG'S RULE: To determine dosage for children ages 1 to 12, you would: divide the child's age in years by the age in years + 12 and multiply by the adult dose. Use ratio and proportion, the Formula Method, or Dimensional Analysis to determine the amount to give.

Example: The physician prescribed milk of magnesia for an 8-year-old patient. The normal adult dose is 30 mL.

Use Young's Rule: Pediatric dose $= \dfrac{\text{age (in years)}}{\text{age (in years)} + 12}$

$\times$ normal adult dose

Pediatric dose $= \dfrac{8}{8 + 12}$

$= \dfrac{8}{20} = \dfrac{2}{5_1} \times \overset{6}{\cancel{30}} \text{ mL} = 12 \text{ mL}$

Answer: 12 mL

Example: A physician prescribed Benadryl elixir for a 4-year-old. The normal adult dose is 25 mg every 4 to 6 hours. Benadryl elixir is available as 12.5 mg/5 mL.

Use Young's Rule: Pediatric dose $= \dfrac{\text{age (in years)}}{\text{age (in years)} + 12}$

$\times$ normal adult dose

Pediatric dose $= \dfrac{4}{4 + 12} = \dfrac{4}{16}$

$= \dfrac{1}{4} \times 25 \text{ mg} = 6.25 \text{ mg}$

Use Ratio and Proportion

6.25 mg : x mL :: 12.5 mg : 5 mL

$12.5x = 5 \times 6.25$

$12.5x = 31.25$

$x = 2.5$ mL

Answer: 2.5 mL

Use the Formula Method

$\dfrac{D}{H} \times Q = $ amount to give

$\dfrac{6.25 \text{ mg}}{12.5 \text{ mL}} \times \text{mL} = 2.5 \text{ mL}$

Answer: 2.5 mL

Use Dimensional Analysis

$x \text{ mL} = \dfrac{5 \text{ mL}}{12.5 \text{ mg}} \times \dfrac{6.25 \text{ mg}}{1}$

$x \text{ mL} = \dfrac{31.25}{12.5} = \dfrac{5}{2} = 2.5 \text{ mL}$

Answer: 2.5 mL

Calculate Dosages Using Rule Based on Weight

> **CLARK'S RULE:** To determine dosage for 2-year-olds and older children, you would: divide the child's weight in pounds by 150 and multiply by the normal adult dose. Use ratio and proportion, the Formula Method, or Dimensional Analysis to determine the amount to give.

Example: The physician prescribed Benadryl elixir for a 4-year-old who weighs about 30 pounds. The normal adult dose is 25 mg every 4 to 6 hours. Benadryl elixir is available as 12.5 mg/5 mL.

Use Clark's Rule: Pediatric dose = $\dfrac{\text{weight in pounds}}{150}$

$\times$ normal adult dose

Pediatric dose = $\dfrac{30}{150} = \dfrac{1}{5}$

$\dfrac{1}{5} \times 25 \text{ mg} = 5 \text{ mg}$

Use Ratio and Proportion

12.5 mg : 5 mL :: 5 mg : x mL

$12.5x = 25$

$x = 2 \text{ mL}$

Answer: 2 mL

Use the Formula Method

$\dfrac{\text{D}}{\text{H}} \times \text{Q} = $ amount to give

$\dfrac{5 \text{ mg}}{12.5 \text{ mg}} \times 5 \text{ mL} = \dfrac{25}{12.5} = 2 \text{ mL}$

Answer: 2 mL

Use Dimensional Analysis

$x \text{ mL} = \dfrac{5 \text{ mL}}{12.5 \text{ mg}} \times \dfrac{5 \text{ mg}}{1}$

$$x \text{ mL} = \frac{5 \times 5}{12.5} = \frac{25}{12.5} = 2 \text{ mL}$$

Answer: 2 mL

Calculate Dosages Using Rule Based on Body Surface Area

Basing a pediatric dosage on BSA is the most accurate way of determining the amount of drug to give. BSA compares a child's weight and height against an average. A nomogram can be used to help estimate BSA (Fig. 15.1).

> **RULE: To determine a pediatric dosage based on BSA, you would: divide the child's BSA in square meters (m²) (use Figure 15.1)* by 1.73 m² (surface area of an average adult) and multiply by the adult dose.**

Example: The physician prescribed Benadryl for an 8-year-old child who weighs 75 pounds and is 50 inches tall (4 feet, 2 inches). The normal adult dose is 25 mg, q.i.d. The nurse would give _____ mg, q.i.d.

(text continues on page 270)

---

*The nomogram is used to determine body surface area. To use the nomograms in Figure 15.1, you need to draw a straight line from the patient's height to his or her weight. You will intersect the surface area column at a number that indicates the patient's body surface area in square meters (m²) (see page 269).

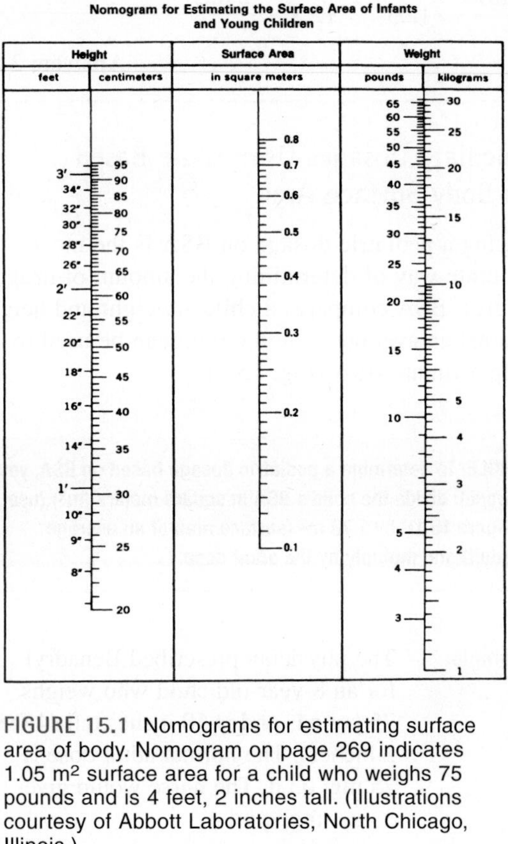

FIGURE 15.1 Nomograms for estimating surface area of body. Nomogram on page 269 indicates 1.05 m² surface area for a child who weighs 75 pounds and is 4 feet, 2 inches tall. (Illustrations courtesy of Abbott Laboratories, North Chicago, Illinois.)

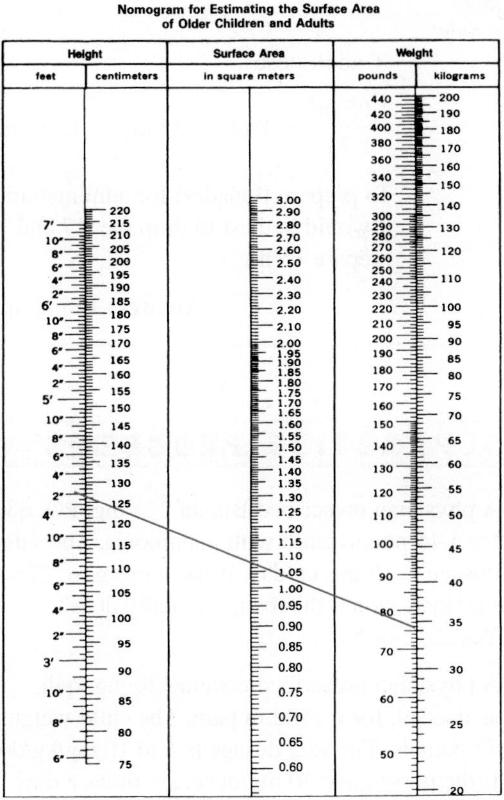
Nomogram for Estimating the Surface Area
of Older Children and Adults
Height
feet
centimeters
Surface Area
in square meters
Weight
pounds
kilograms

FIGURE 15.1 (continued)

Use Body
Surface
Area Rule:

$$\frac{\text{child's surface area in square meters (m}^2)}{1.73 \text{ m}^2}$$

$\times$ adult dose

$$\frac{1.05 \text{ m}^2}{1.73} = 0.60 \times 25 \text{ mg} = 15.17 \text{ mg}$$

To prepare Benadryl for administration, it would be best to drop the .17 and prepare 15 mg.

Answer: 15 mg, q.i.d.

PRACTICE PROBLEMS

1. A physician prescribed Biaxin 275 mg, PO, q8h, for a 44-pound child with pneumonia. The safe dosage is 15 mg/kg/day. If the nurse gave 275 mg/dose, would this be a safe daily dose? Yes _____ or No _____

2. A physician prescribed codeine 30 mg, q4h, as needed, for a child in pain. The child weighs 44 pounds. The safe dosage is 5 to 10 mg/kg/dose. If the nurse gave 30 mg/dose, six times a day, would this be a safe dose? Yes _____ or No _____

3. An emergency department physician ordered Valium 4 mg, IV, stat, for a 44-pound child with a seizure. The safe dosage range is 0.04 to 0.2 mg/kg/dose. The nurse gave _____ mg. Is this a safe dose? Yes _____ or No _____

4. The physician ordered Augmentin Suspension 550 mg, PO, q8h, for a child with otitis media. Augmentin is labeled 250 mg/5 mL. The nurse would administer _____ mL/8 hr.

5. The physician prescribed Macrobid 200 mg, PO, q6h, for an 88-pound child. The child weighs _____ kg. The safe dosage range is 5 to 7 mg/kg/day. Therefore, the safe dosage range for this child is _____ mg/dose. If the nurse gave 200 mg/dose, would this be a safe dose? Yes _____ or No _____

6. The physician prescribed nafcillin 1 gram, q6h, for a 132-pound teenager. The teenager weighs _____ kg. The safe dosage range is 50 to 100 mg/kg/day. Therefore, the safe dosage range for this teenager is _____ mg/dose. If the nurse gave 1 gram/dose, would this be safe? Yes _____ or No _____

7. A physician ordered penicillin V potassium 375 mg, PO, q6h, for a 66-pound child. The child weighs _____ kg. The safe dosage range is 25 to 50 mg/kg/24 hr. The dosage range for this child is _____ mg/dose. Is this a safe dose? Yes _____ or No _____

8. A physician prescribed Dilantin 50 mg, PO, q12h, for a 33-pound child with a seizure disorder. The child weighs _____ kg. The safe dosage range is 5 to 10 mg/kg/day. The dosage range for this child is _____ mg/dose. Is this a safe dose? Yes _____ or No _____

9. A physician ordered Orapred Liquid 20 mg, PO, q12h, for a 44-pound child. The child weighs _____ kg. The safe dosage range is 0.5 to 2 mg/kg/day. The safe dosage range for this child is _____ mg/dose. Orapred Liquid is labeled as 5 mg/mL. The nurse would give _____ mL/dose. Is this a safe dose? Yes _____ or No _____

10. The physician ordered ranitidine HCL 15 mg, PO, q12h, for a 5-kg infant with GERD. The safe dosage range is 5 to 10 mg/kg/day. The safe dosage range for this child is _____ mg/dose. If the nurse gave 30 mg/day, would this be a safe dose? Yes _____ or No _____

11. A physician prescribed Accutane 50 mg, PO, twice a day, for acne for a 110-pound teenager. The safe dosage range is 0.5 to 2 mg/kg/day. The safe dosage range for this teenager is _____ mg/dose. If the nurse gave 100 mg/dose, would this be a safe dose? Yes _____ or No _____

12. The physician prescribed Tylenol drops 100 mg, PO, q4h, p.r.n. for temperature greater than 101.4°F for an infant who weighs 8 kg. Tylenol drops are available as 80 mg/0.8 mL. The safe dosage range is 10 to 15 mg/kg/dose. The dosage range for this infant is _____ mg. The nurse would give _____ mL of Tylenol. Is this a safe dose? Yes _____ or No _____

13. The physician prescribed Ceclor 200 mg, PO, every 8 hours, for a 33-pound toddler. The safe dosage range is 20 to 40 mg/kg/day. The dosage range for this toddler is _____ mg to _____ mg. Is this a safe dose? Yes _____ or No _____

> ✓ **Critical Thinking Check:**
>
> If the physician increased the dosage of Ceclor
> to 300 mg/8 hr, would the dosage be within a
> safe range to give? _____ **Yes or No?**

14. A 4-year-old is prescribed one dose of
    Rocephin 300 mg, IM. The label on the vial is
    Rocephin 500 mg/2.5 mL. You will administer
    _____ mL.

15. Using BSA, calculate a physician order of
    Tylenol drops for a 6-year-old who weighs 42
    pounds and is 45 inches tall (3 feet, 9 inches).
    The normal adult dose is 650 mg. The nurse
    would administer _____ mg each dose.
    Tylenol drops are available as labeled 80 mg/0.8
    mL. The nurse would administer _____ mL.

Calculate Pediatric Flow Rate

A volume-controlled infusion device or a Buretrol or
Soluset is always used for pediatric intravenous therapy. An electronic pump or controller is also almost
always used to regulate the infusion. IV tubing with
a drop factor of 60 gtt/mL is recommended (required
for infants and small children) because the amount of
IV volume is less than that prescribed for adults. The
guidelines for regulating flow rate and mL/hr, using a
pump or controller, are the same for a child as for an
adult. However, the rates must be closely monitored
to prevent fluid overload.

Example: Give 200 mL of D5LR over 4 hours to a 5-year-old child. An IV pump is used.

Use This Formula:

$$\frac{\text{total volume}}{\text{total time (minutes)}} = \frac{x \text{ (mL/hr)}}{60 \text{ minutes}}$$

$$\frac{200 \text{ mL}}{240 \text{ min}} = \frac{x \text{ (mL/hr)}}{60 \text{ min}}$$

$$240x = 12,000$$

$$x = \frac{12,000}{240}$$

$$x = 50 \text{ mL/hr}$$

Answer: Set pump to deliver 50 mL/hr.

Calculate Intravenous Medication Dosages

Dosages for IV medications are calculated on mg/kg. Always refer to a pediatric reference to determine the safe dosage range for medications. Some institutions provide standard guidelines to assist the nurse in preparing IV pediatric dosages. *Remember* that most drugs are administered in a small amount of diluent with the average volume of solutions being between 10 and 20 mL for infants and smaller children.

The primary caution in administering IV medications to pediatric patients is the amount of *fluid volume* that is used. It is essential that pediatric intravenous therapy be as exact as possible because infants and children have a narrow range of fluid balance. Therefore, Buretrols (Solusets) and other volume-controlled infusion devices (electronic pumps or controllers) are almost always used to regulate the infusion. These control devices reduce the possibility of fluid overload. Syringe pumps can also be used to deliver IV medications. Always *remember* when administering IV medications that the total fluid volume consists of medication diluent volume, IV solution volume, and flush volume (5–15 mL). See Figure 15.2.

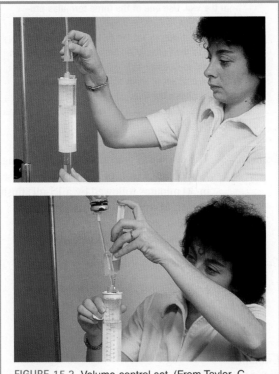

FIGURE 15.2   Volume-control set. (From Taylor, C., Lillis, C., and LeMone, P. [2001]. *Fundamentals of nursing: The art and science of nursing care* [5th ed.]. Philadelphia: Lippincott Williams & Wilkins, p. 645.)

> **RULE: To give pediatric intravenous medications, you would:**
> - Convert the child's weight to kilograms
> - Estimate safe dosage range using a recommended reference
> - Calculate total amount of medication to be given over 24 hours
> - Determine the amount of drug to be withdrawn from the vial. Use one of the three formulas presented earlier.
> - Select the gtt/min to set the IV. Use Dimensional Analysis or the Formula Method to calculate gtt/min (presented in Chapter 10).
> - Know the amount of flush solution that is recommended to flush the line

Example: The physician prescribed Kefzol 125 mg, IV, q6h, in 50 mL of D51/4 NS to infuse in 30 minutes followed by a 15-mL flush. The child weighs 44 pounds. Kefzol is available as 250 mg. Safe IV dosage range is 25 to 50 mg/kg/day.

Convert: 44 pounds to kilograms

Use: 1 kg : 2.2 lbs :: x kg : 44 lbs

$2.2x = 44$

$x = 44 \div 2.2 = 20$ kg

Estimate Safe Dosage Range:
- 25 mg : 1 kg :: x mg : 20 kg

$x = 25 \times 20$

$x = 500$ mg

- 50 mg : 1 kg :: x mg : 20 kg

    $x = 50 \times 20$

    $x = 1,000$ mg

Determine 24-Hour Total:

Safe dosage range is 500 to 1,000 mg/day. A physician prescribed 125 mg, q6h (4 times/day), which equals 500 mg/day. This amount falls within the safe dosage range.

Determine Amount of Drug:

Use $\dfrac{D}{H} \times Q = x$

125 mg : x mL :: 250 mg : 2 mL (volume added to vial)

$250x = 250$

$x = 1$ mL to be withdrawn from the vial

Calculate gtt/min:

Use this formula:

$$\dfrac{\text{total volume} \times \text{drop factor}}{\text{total time in minutes}} = \text{gtt/min}$$

49 mL of solution (+) 1 mL of medication (+)

15 mL of flush $\times$ 60 (drop factor)/ 30 minutes

$$= \dfrac{65 \text{ mL } (49 + 1 + 15) \times 60 \text{ gtt}}{30 \text{ minutes}}$$

$= 130$ gtt/min

Answer: 130 gtt/min

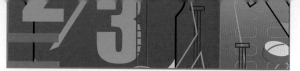

End of Chapter Review

1. The physician prescribed Orapred 10 mg, PO, every 12 hours, for a 22-pound child. The safe dosage range is 0.5 to 2.0 mg/kg/day. The dosage range for this child is _____ mg/dose. This is/is not within a safe range. _____

2. The physician prescribed Spectrobid 25 mg/kg for a 22-pound 12-month-old. The medicine was to be given q12h. The child would receive _____ mg every 12 hours.

3. A physician prescribed Pen-Vee K for an 18-month-old. The medicine comes in a powder for oral suspension, 250 mg/5 mL. The normal adult dose is 250 mg every 6 hours. The nurse would give _____ mg in _____ mL every 6 hours.

4. The physician prescribed Benadryl to relieve itching from chicken pox for an 8-year-old. Benadryl comes in an elixir of 12.5 mg/5 mL. The normal adult dose is 25 mg every 12 hours as needed. The nurse would give _____ mg in _____ mL every 12 hours.

5. A physician prescribed Dimetane for a 30-pound child. The drug comes as an elixir, 2 mg/5 mL. The normal adult dose is 4.0 mg every 4 to 6 hours. The nurse would give _____ mg in _____ mL every 4 to 6 hours.

6. A physician prescribed Phenergan for preoperative medication for a 44-pound child. Phenergan is to be given as 1 mg/kg of body weight. The nurse would give _____ mg preoperatively.

7. A physician prescribed Keflex 150 mg, PO, q6h. The child weighs 33 pounds. Keflex is labeled 125 mg/5 mL. The safe dosage range is 25 to 50 mg/kg/day. The child's weight is _____ kg; the safe dosage range for this child per day is _____. The child should receive _____ mL/q6h. This is/is not within a safe range. _____

8. A physician prescribed phenobarbital 50 mg/q12h for a 66-pound child. The safe dosage range is 3 to 5 mg/kg/day. The child's weight is _____ kg; the safe dosage range for this child/day is _____. The child should receive _____ /day. This is/is not within a safe range. _____

> ### Critical Thinking Check:
>
> If the child gains 4 pounds, would the dosage per day be within a safe range to give? _____
> **Yes or No?**

9. A 10-year-old is ordered a stat dose of morphine sulfate IV for pain. The child weighs 90 pounds and is 52 inches tall (4 feet, 4 inches). Calculate the dosage to administer using a BSA of 1.22 m². The normal adult dose of morphine sulfate is 10 mg. You should administer _____ mg of morphine sulfate. Morphine sulfate is available in 10 mg/2 mL. You would administer _____ mL.

10. A physician prescribed Pelamine for a 7-year-old who weighs 70 pounds and is 50 inches tall. The

normal adult dose is 50 mg every 6 hours. Refer to the nomogram in Figure 15.1 to find the child's surface area in square meters. Determine the BSA. Calculate the dosage the child should receive in four equally divided doses. _____

11. The physician prescribed 20 mg of Demerol, every 6 hours postoperatively, to a 7-year-old child who weighs 20 kg. Demerol is available as 25 mg/mL. You would give _____ mL/6 hr.

12. The physician prescribed 5 mg of Garamycin for a child. The medication is available as 20 mg/2 mL. To give 5 mg, you would give _____ mL.

13. The physician prescribed metronidazole suspension 325 mg, PO, q12h, for a 44-kg child. The safe dosage is 15 mg/kg/day. The nurse would give _____ mg/day. Is this a safe dose? Yes ___ or No____. Metronidazole suspension is available as 50 mg/mL. The nurse would give ____ mL/dose.

14. The physician prescribed amoxicillin suspension 225 mg, PO, q8h, for a 33-pound child. The safe dosage range is 25 to 50 mg/kg/day. The safe dosage range for this child is _____ mg/dose. Is this a safe dose? Yes _____ or No_____

15. The physician prescribed caffeine citrate 30 mg, PO, once a day for an 11-pound infant. The safe dosage range is 5 to 10 mg/kg/dose. Is this a safe dose? Yes _____ or No_____

16. The physician prescribed Ceclor 300 mg, PO, q8h, for a 66-pound child. The safe dosage range is 20 to 40 mg/kg/day. The safe dosage

range for this child is _____ mg/dose. Is this a
safe dose? Yes _____ or No _____

17. The physician prescribed chloral hydrate 400
mg, PO, for one dose for an 11-pound infant
prior to an EEG study. The safe dosage range is
25 to 50 mg/kg/dose. Is this a safe dose? Yes
_____ or No _____

18. The physician prescribed Aldactone 20 mg, PO,
q12h, for a 33-pound child. The safe dosage
range is 1 to 3.3 mg/kg/24 hr. The safe dosage
range for this child is _____ mg/dose. Is this a
safe dose? Yes _____ or No _____

19. The physician prescribed Depakene 1 gram, PO,
q12h, for an 88-pound child. The safe dosage
range is 30 to 60 mg/kg/day. The safe dosage
range for this child is _____ mg/dose. The nurse
would give _____ mg/dose. Is this a safe dose?
Yes _____ or No _____

20. The physician prescribed Lasix 5 mg, PO, every
morning, for an 11-pound infant with a cardiac
problem. The safe dosage range is 0.5 to 2 mg/kg/
day. The safe dosage range for this child is _____
mg/dose. Lasix liquid is labeled 10 mg/mL. The
nurse would give _____ mL each morning. Is this
a safe dose? Yes _____ or No _____

21. The physician prescribed gentamicin 12 mg,
IV, q8h, for an infant who weighs 6 kg. The safe
dosage range is 2.5 mg/kg/dose. Gentamicin is
available as 20 mg/mL. You would administer
_____ mL, q8h. This is/is not a safe
dose. _____

22. The physician prescribed morphine sulfate 5 mg, IV, q2h, p.r.n. for pain for a child who weighs 88 pounds. The safe dosage range is 0.05 to 0.2 mg/kg/dose. Morphine sulfate is available as 15 mg/1 mL. The child's weight is _____ kg; the safe dosage range for this child is _____. The child should receive _____ mL IV. This is/is not within a safe range. _____

23. The physician prescribed vancomycin 300 mg, IV, q6h, for a 66-pound child. The safe dosage range is 40 mg/kg/day. The child's weight is _____ kg; the safe dosage range for this child is _____. This child should receive _____ mg IV, q6h. This is/is not within a safe range. _____

24. The physician prescribed Lasix 40 mg, IV, stat, for an 88-pound child. The label reads, "Lasix, 10 mg/mL." The safe dosage range is 0.5 to 2.0 mg/kg/dose. The child's weight is _____ kg; the safe dosage range for this child is _____. This child should receive _____ mL. This is/is not within a safe range. _____

25. The physician prescribed ampicillin 250 mg in 30 mL of D5/0.22% NSS to infuse over 30 minutes, followed by a 15-mL flush. Ampicillin requires 5 mL for reconstitution. The drop factor is 60 gtt/mL. The pump or controller should be set at _____ mL/hr.

26. The physician prescribed Rocephin 500 mg in 50 mL of NSS to infuse over 30 minutes via a Buretrol, followed by a 15-mL flush. Rocephin

requires 10 mL for reconstitution. The nurse should set the controller at _____ mL/hr.

27. The physician prescribed gentamicin 10 mg in 50 mL of D5/0.45% NSS to infuse over 30 minutes via a Buretrol, followed by a 15-mL flush. The drop factor is 60 gtt/mL. Gentamicin is available as 20 mg/2 mL. You should set the rate at _____ mL/hr.

28. A child is to receive an IV medication of 75 mg/3 mL diluted to 55 mL using NSS. The IV is to infuse over 45 minutes, followed by a 15-mL flush. A microdrip Soluset is used. The nurse should set the pump at _____ mL/hr.

29. A child is to receive Dilantin 25 mg/2 mL diluted to 10 mL using NSS. The IV is to infuse over 10 minutes via a microdrip Buretrol, followed by a 10-mL flush. The nurse should set the pump at _____ mL/hr.

30. A child is to receive 1 gram/4 mL of an antibiotic. The medication is to be diluted in 60 mL of D5/1/4 NSS and to infuse over 60 minutes, followed by a 15-mL flush. It is a microdrop tubing. The Buretrol is on a pump that should be set at _____ mL/hr.

31. A child is to receive 30 mL of an intravenous solution every hour through a volume control set that delivers 60 microdrops/mL. The flow rate should be set at _____ gtt/min to deliver 30 mL/hr.

32. Give a child aminophylline 250 mg IVPB in 50 mL of NSS over 1 hour via a Buretrol that delivers 60 microdrops/mL, followed by a

10-mL flush. Aminophylline is available in 250 mg/10 mL. You would give _____ gtt/min with a total volume of _____ mL.

33. The physician prescribed Solu-Medrol 20 mg by slow IV push for an asthmatic child. Solu-Medrol is labeled 40 mg/mL. The nurse would give _____ mL over 3 minutes.

34. An infant is to receive 15 mL of D5/0.22% NSS solution every hour through a volume control set that delivers 60 microdrops/mL. The flow rate should be set at _____ gtt/min to deliver 15 mL/hr.

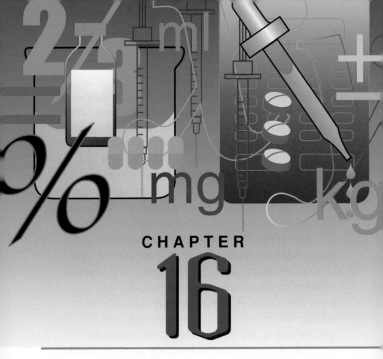

Solutions

LEARNING OBJECTIVES

After completing this chapter, you should be able to:

- Calculate the reconstitution of medications packaged as powders and both single- and double-strength parenteral solutions.
- Calculate the reconstitution of an oral or parenteral feeding.
- Calculate the preparation of a topical or irrigating solution from (a) a solution, (b) a pure drug, and (c) a stock solution.

Solutions are mixtures of liquids, solids, or gases (known as *solutes*) that are dissolved in a diluent (known as a *solvent*). Solutions can be administered externally (e.g., compresses, soaks, irrigations) or internally (e.g., parenteral medications, nutritional formulas).

Solutions can be prepared from full-strength drugs or from stock solutions. Full-strength drugs are considered to be 100% pure, whereas stock solutions contain drugs in a given solution strength, always less than 100%, from which weaker solutions are made. Solution strengths can be expressed in a percentage or ratio format; for example, a 1/2-strength solution means that there is one part solute to two parts total solution. *Remember:* the *less* solvent added, the *greater* the solution strength, and the *more* solvent added, the *weaker* the solution strength.

Solution problems are basically problems involving percents that can be solved using the ratio and proportion method. When setting up the ratio and proportion for a solution made from a pure drug or from a stock solution, *use the strength of the desired solution to the strength of the available solution as one ratio, and the solute to the solution as the other ratio.* desired solution strength : available solution strength :: amount of solute : total amount of solution.

You can substitute the Formula Method when using a proportion for a solution made from a stock solution:

$$\frac{\text{Desired strength}}{\text{Available strength}} \times \text{total amount of solution}$$

$$= \text{amount of solute needed}$$

$$\frac{D}{H} \times Q = x$$

When calculating solution problems, it is important to remember two things:

1. Work within the same measurement system (e.g., milligrams with milliliters, grains with minims).
2. Change solutions expressed in the fraction or colon format to a percent (1:2 or 1/2 is equal to 50%).

Reconstitution: Preparing Injectable Medications Packaged as Powders

Some drugs are unstable in solution so they are packaged as a powder. When the *available amount of a drug* is in a solute form (dry powder), the drug needs to be dissolved or reconstituted by adding a liquid diluent (solvent). The drug label or package insert will list directions for adding the diluent and mixing thoroughly. Diluents must always be sterile when added to a dry powder. Sample diluents would include:

- Bacteriostatic water
- Special packaged diluent
- 5% dextrose solution
- Sodium chloride (0.9%)
- Sterile water

Reconstituted parenteral medications are available in *single-strength* (either single- or multiple-dose vials) or *multiple-strength* solutions. *Remember:* For multiple-strength solutions, *the dosage strength depends on the amount of diluent;* for example, 75 mL of diluent may yield a solution of 200,000 U/mL, whereas 30 mL of diluent may yield 500,000 U/mL.

Basic Steps for Reconstitution

Remember: always read the package insert or labeled directions for reconstitution very carefully because directions will vary. Follow these steps:

- *Read* specific directions for reconstitution.
- *Note* length of time medication will remain stable after reconstitution.
- *Select* type and quantity of recommended diluent.
- *Estimate* reconstituted dosage.
- *Note* total dosage volume. Reconstituted solutions will always exceed the volume of the added diluent.
- *Determine* the number of doses available in the vial.
- *Label* medications with the date and time of preparation and expiration and reconstituted dosage if using a multiple-dose vial. *Note:* some preparations allow for different quantities of diluent, which result in different solution strengths.
- *Initial* labeled vials.
- *Use* one of the three methods to calculate dosages.

Note: if you choose to use ratio and proportion, *what you have is the dosage strength after mixing the drug.* If you choose to use Dimensional Analysis, the *dosage strength is used as the first fraction.*

Single-Strength Parenteral Solutions

Example: Give 250 mg of Ancef, IM, every 8 hours. The medication is available as a powder in a 1-gram vial.

Reconstitute: Labeled directions: Reconstitute by adding 2.5 mL of sterile water for

injection. Shake well until dissolved.
Solution concentration will equal
330 mg per mL. Fluid volume will equal
3.0 mL.

Dissolve 1 gram of powder with 2.5 mL
of sterile water.

Use Ratio and Proportion

250 mg : x mL :: 1,000 mg : 3 mL

$1,000x = 750$

$$x = \frac{750}{1,000} = \frac{3 \text{ mL}}{4}$$

Answer: 0.75 mL

Use the Formula Method

$$\frac{D}{H} \times Q = x$$

$$\frac{250 \text{ mg}}{^*1,000 \text{ mg}} = \frac{1}{4}$$

$$\frac{1}{4} \times 3.0 \text{ mL} = 0.75 \text{ mL or } \frac{3}{4}$$

Answer: 0.75 mL

Use Dimensional Analysis

$$x \text{ mL} = \frac{3 \text{ mL}}{1,000 \text{ mg}} \times \frac{250 \text{ mg}}{1}$$

$$x \text{ mL} = \frac{750}{1,000} = \frac{3 \text{ mL}}{4}$$

Answer: 0.75 mL

Example: Give 125 mg of Solu-Medrol, IM.
Medication is available as a powder in a
500-mg vial.

Reconstitute: Labeled directions: Reconstitute by
adding 8 mL of sterile water for injection. Solution concentration will equal
62.5 mg per mL. Fluid volume will
equal >8 mL.

Dissolve 500 mg of powder with 8 mL
of sterile water.

Use Ratio and Proportion

125 mg : x mL :: 500 mg : 8 mL

$500x = 1,000$

$x = 2$ mL

Answer: 2 mL

Use the Formula Method

$$\frac{D}{H} \times Q = x$$

$$\frac{125 \text{ mg}}{500 \text{ mg}} = \frac{1}{4} \times 8 \text{ mL} = 2 \text{ mL}$$

Answer: 2 mL

Use Dimensional Analysis

$$x \text{ mL} = \frac{8 \text{ mL}}{500 \text{ mg}} \times \frac{125 \text{ mg}}{1}$$

$$x \text{ mL} = \frac{1,000}{500} = 2 \text{ mL}$$

Answer: 2 mL

Multiple-Strength Parenteral Solutions

Example: Give Geopen 1 g, IM. Medication is available as a powder in a 2-g vial.

Reconstitute: Labeled directions: Reconstitute by adding 4 mL of sterile water for IM injection (8 mL is required for IV use). Solution concentration (g/mL) will vary with mL of diluent added.

For example:

4 mL of diluent = 1 g/2.5 mL

5 mL of diluent = 1 g/3 mL

7.2 mL of diluent = 1 g/4 mL

Use the Formula Method

$$\frac{D}{H} = \frac{1 \text{ g}}{1 \text{ g/2.5 mL}}$$

Answer: 2.5 mL

Preparing an Oral or Enteral Feeding

Frequently oral and enteral feedings are packaged as ordered. However, sometimes the feeding solution needs to be prepared from a powder or a liquid concentrate. Sterile water or tap water is normally used to dilute nutritional formulas.

Example: Give 300 mL of 1/3 strength Sustacal every 6 hours through an NG tube. Sustacal is available in a 10-ounce can.

Estimate	A 10-ounce can of Sustacal
Available	equals 300 mL.
mL:	(10 ounces × 30 mL = 300 mL)

Calculate:	1/3 strength = 1/3 solute concentration:
	1/3 × 300 mL = 100 mL solute

Prepare:	100 mL of Sustacal diluted in 200 mL
	of solvent is needed every 6 hours.

Answer: Add 200 mL of water to 100 mL of Sustacal to prepare 1/3-strength feeding.

Preparing Topical and Irrigating Solutions

Preparing a Solution From a Solution or Pure Drug

Example: Prepare 500 mL of a 5% boric acid solution from pure boric acid crystals.

Use the Formula Method

$$\frac{D}{H} \times Q = x$$

$$\frac{5\%}{100\%} = \frac{50}{100} = \frac{1}{20}$$

$$\frac{1}{20} \times 500 \text{ mL} = 25 \text{ g}$$

Answer: 25 grams; weigh and dissolve 25 grams in 500 mL of water.*

---

*The answer is in grams because the solid form of boric acid was used and the solution desired was expressed in metric units.

Example: Prepare 1.0 liter of a 10% solution from a pure drug.

Use the Formula Method

$$\frac{D}{H} \times Q = x$$

$$\frac{10\%}{100\%} = \frac{10}{100} = \frac{1}{10}$$

$$\frac{1}{10} \times 1,000 \text{ mL} = 100 \text{ mL}$$

> **Answer:** 100 mL; measure 100 mL of pure drug and add 900 mL of water to prepare 1.0 liter of a 10% solution.

Preparing a Solution From a Stock Solution

Example: Prepare 250 mL of a 5% solution from a 50% solution.

Use the Formula Method

$$\frac{D}{H} \times Q = x$$

$$\frac{5\%}{50\%_1} \times 250^5 \text{ mL} = 25 \text{ mL of solute needed}$$

> **Answer:** The solution has a ratio strength of 1:10. Measure 25 mL of solute and add 225 mL of water to prepare 250 mL.

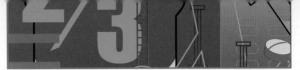

End of Unit 3 Review

Complete the following problems:

1. To prepare 400 mL of a 2% sodium bicarbonate solution from pure drug, you would need _____ grams of solute.

2. To make 1.5 L of a 5.0% solution from a 25% solution, you would need _____ mL of solute. Add _____ mL of water to make 1.5 L.

3. There is 500 mL of 40% magnesium sulfate solution available for a soak. To make a 30% solution, you would need _____ mL of solute. Add _____ mL of water to make 500 mL.

4. The physician prescribed 500 mg of Cefizox, IM, every 12 hours, for a genitourinary infection. The medication is available as a powder in a 2-gram vial. Reconstitute it with 6.0 mL of sterile water for injection and shake well. Solution concentration will provide 270 mg/mL. Fluid volume will equal 7.4 mL. Use approximate quantities for dosage calculations. Give _____ mL every 12 hours.

5. Methicillin sodium 1.5 grams, IM, was prescribed for a systemic infection. Four (4) grams of the medication is available as a powder in a vial. Directions state to reconstitute it with 5.7 mL of sterile water for injection and shake well. Solution concentration will provide 500 mg/mL. To give 1.5 grams, the nurse would give _____ mL.

6. The physician prescribed 125 mg of Solu-Medrol, IM, for severe inflammation. The medication is available as a powder in a 0.5-gram vial. Reconstitute it according to directions so that each 8 mL will contain 0.5 grams of Solu-Medrol. The nurse would then give _____ mL to give 125 mg.

End of Unit 3 Review

Solve the following drug administration problems and reduce each answer to its lowest terms.

1. Give 1.5 grams. The drug is available in 250-mg tablets. Give _____ tablet(s).

2. Give 2 teaspoons. The drug is available as 250 mg/ 5 mL. Give _____ mg.

3. Give 600 mg. The drug is available in 200-mg tablets. Give _____ tablet(s).

4. Give 0.3 grams. The drug is available as 150 mg/ 2.5 mL. Give _____ mL.

5. Give 75 mg. The drug is available as 25 mg/ teaspoon. Give _____ mL.

> **Critical Thinking Check:**
>
> Would it seem logical to give a tablespoon of medication to give 75 mg? _____ **Yes or No?**

6. Give 125 mg. The drug is available in 0.25-gram tablets. Give _____ tablet(s).

7. Give gr 1/100. The drug is available in 60-mg tablets. Give _____ tablet(s).

8. Give a liquid medication to a 6-month-old. The drug is available as 100 mg/5 mL for the normal adult daily dose. Give _____ mL/day.

9. Give 50 mg. The drug is available as 100 mg/ 2 mL. Give _____ mL.

10. Give 0.75 mg. The drug is available as 500 mcg/ 2 mL. Give _____ mL.

11. Give gr iii. The drug is available as 60 mg/mL. Give _____ mL.

12. Give gr 1/8. The drug is available as 15 mg/mL. Give _____ mL.

13. Give 0.3 mg. The drug is available as 200 mcg/ mL. Give _____ mL.

14. Give gr 1/6. The drug is available as 8 mg/mL. Give _____ mL.

15. Give 0.25 grams. The drug is available as 300 mg/ 2 mL. Give _____ mL.

16. Give 500 mg of a medication that is available as a powder in a 2-gram vial. Reconstitute it by adding 11.5 mL of sterile water for injection. Each 1.5 mL of solution contains 250 mg of the medication. Give _____ mL.

17. Give 1 gram of a medication that is available as a powder in a 2-gram vial. Reconstitute it by adding 5 mL to achieve a concentration of 330 mg/mL. Give _____ mL.

18. Give 125 mg of a drug dissolved in 100 mL of a solution over 30 minutes. You would give _____ mL/hr.

19. Give 1,000 mL of a solution over 8 hours, using a drop factor of 10 gtt/mL. Give _____ gtt/min.

Critical Thinking Check:

If the available tubing had a drop factor of 15 gtt/mL, would you expect the gtt/min to be greater or less than the gtt/min for a drop factor of 10? _____ **Greater or Less?**

---

20. Give 500 mL of a solution over 10 hours, using a drop factor of 60 gtt/mL. Give _____ gtt/min.

21. Give 1,000 mL of a solution over 6 hours, using a drop factor of 15 gtt/mL. Give _____ gtt/min.

22. Give 800 mL of a solution at 12 gtt/min, using a drop factor of 10 gtt/mL. Give over _____ hours and _____ minutes.

23. Give 250 mg of a solution in 500 mL at 10 mL/hr. Give _____ mg/hr or _____ mcg/min.

24. Give 15 units of U-100 Regular insulin by subcutaneous injection. Use U-100 Regular insulin and a U-100 syringe. Draw up insulin in the syringe to the _____ unit marking.

25. Give 35 units of NPH and 10 units of Regular insulin, using U-100 insulins and syringes. Draw up _____ units of _____ first, followed by _____ units of _____.

26. Give 2,500 units of heparin subcutaneously. Vial concentration is 5,000 units/mL. Give _____ mL.

27. Give 1,000 mL of D5W with 15,000 units of heparin to infuse at 30 mL/hr. Give _____ units/hr.

28. Give 800 units/hr of heparin IV. Consider that 500 mL of D5W is available, with 20,000 units of heparin added. The drop factor is 60 gtt/min. Give _____ gtt/min.

29. Give 1,000 mL of D5W with 40,000 units of heparin to infuse at 25 mL/hr. Give _____ units/hr, which *is* or *is not* a safe dose. _____

30. Give 0.5 mL of IPV vaccine subcutaneously. A 5-mL multiple-dose vial is available. Give _____ mL. The vial contains a total of _____ doses.

31. An ER physician ordered Toradol 30 mg, IV, stat, for a 154-pound teenager that had a tibia fracture. The safe dosage range is 0.5 mg/kg/dose, IV/IM. Is this a safe dose? Yes _____ or No _____

32. A physician prescribed Demerol 25 mg, IV, q4h, as needed for pain for a 44-pound child. The safe dosage range is 1 to 1.5 mg/kg/dose. The safe dosage range for this child is _____ mg/dose. Demerol is available as 100 mg/2 mL. The nurse would give _____ mL. Is this a safe dose? Yes _____ or No _____

33. A physician ordered Solu-Medrol 30 mg, IV, q12h, for an 88-pound child. The safe dosage range is 0.5 to 1.7 mg/kg/day. The safe dosage range for this child is _____ mg/dose. Solu-Medrol is available as 40 mg/mL. The nurse

would give _____ mL. Is this a safe dose?
Yes _____ or No _____

34. The physician prescribed gentamicin 15 mg, IV,
    q8h, for a 6.5-kg infant. The safe dosage range
    is 6 to 7.5 mg/kg/day. The safe dosage range for
    this infant is _____ mg/dose. Gentamicin is
    labeled 10 mg/mL for IV use. The nurse would
    give _____ mL. Is this a safe dose? Yes _____
    or No _____

35. The physician prescribed vancomycin 0.4 gram,
    IV, q8h, for a 66-pound child. The safe dosage
    is 40 mg/kg/day. The dosage range for this
    child is _____ mg/dose. The nurse would
    give _____ mg. Is this a safe dose? Yes _____
    or No _____

36. The physician prescribed morphine sulfate 6
    mg, IV, q3h, as needed for pain for a 110-pound
    child. The safe dosage range is 0.1 to 0.2 mg/kg/
    dose. The safe dosage range for this child
    is _____ mg/dose. Morphine is available as
    15 mg/mL. The nurse would give _____ mL.
    Is this a safe dose? Yes _____ or No _____

37. The physician prescribed 1.0 mg, IM, of leu-
    covorin calcium, to be given once a day for
    the treatment of megaloblastic anemia. The
    medication is available as a powder in a
    50-mg vial. Reconstitute it with 5.0 mL of
    bacteriostatic water for injection. Shake it
    well. Solution concentration will yield 10
    mg/mL. Fluid volume will equal 5.0 mL.
    Give _____ mL, once a day.

38. The physician prescribed 25 mg of Librium, IM. Add 2 mL of special diluent to yield 100 mg/ 2 mL. The nurse should give _____ mL.

Answer the next three questions by referring to the corresponding drug labels.

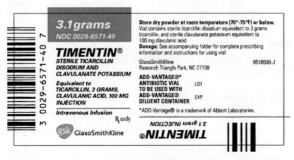

Timentin (Courtesy of GlaxoSmithKline, Philadelphia, PA).

39. The physician prescribed Timentin 3.1 grams, IV, every 6 hours for a patient with a severe infection. The patient would receive _____ g of Timentin in 24 hours.

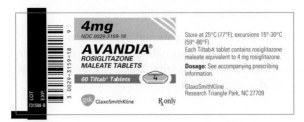

Avandia (Courtesy of GlaxoSmithKline, Philadelphia, PA).

40. The physician prescribed Avandia 8 milligrams twice a day. The patient would receive _____ mg in 24 hours.

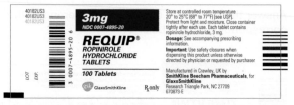

Requip (Courtesy of GlaxoSmithKline, Philadelphia, PA).

41. A patient with Parkinson's disease is to receive Requip, 2 mg, three times a day. The nurse would administer _____ tablet(s) each dose for a total of _____ mg in 24 hours.

42. In order to control a patient's blood glucose, an insulin infusion is prescribed. Insulin 100 units in 100 mL is started at 6 mL/hr. You document that the patient is receiving _____ units/hr.

43. Versed 50 mg in 100 mL is running at 3 mL/hr to manage anxiety in a mechanically ventilated patient. You document that the patient is receiving _____ mg/hr.

44. A patient with sepsis and hypotension is prescribed vasopressin 20 units in 100 mL NSS to start at 0.01 units/min. You would set the pump at _____ mL/hr.

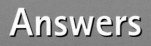

Answers

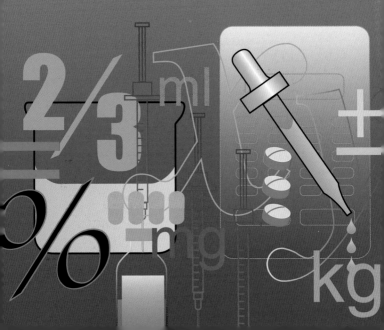

CHAPTER 1: Preassessment Test: Mathematics Skills Review

Basic Math Pretest: Pages 4–9

1. viii
2. xiii
3. ii$\overline{\text{ss}}$
4. xxxvii
5. Li

6. 11 1/2
7. 16
8. 65
9. 9
10. 19

11. 5/8
12. 1/2
13. 1/2
14. 4/15

15. 1/3
16. 1/150
17. 1/100
18. 3/4

19. 3/8
20. 8 2/5
21. 3/4
22. 6 1/8
23. 1/60
24. 3 3/7
25. 1/48
26. 2/5

27. 14/5
28. 27/4
29. 94/9
30. 57/7

31. 3
32. 4 1/18
33. 3 2/11
34. 1 3/13

35. 0.33
36. 0.40
37. 0.37
38. 0.75

39. 1.81
40. 4.00
41. 5.87
42. 2.13

43. 48.78
44. 0.250
45. 72
46. 3.4

47. 1/4
48. 4/5
49. 1/3
50. 9/20
51. 3/4
52. 3/5
53. 3
54. 16
55. 2.6
56. 10
57. 0.75
58. 12
59. 24
60. 0.16
61. 0.9
62. 0.2

63. 20%	64. 36%	65. 7%
66. 12.5%	67. 10.3%	68. 183%
69. 25%	70. 60%	71. 1%
72. 198%	73. 1.2%	74. 14.2%
75. 0.25	76. 0.40	77. 0.80
78. 0.15	79. 0.048	80. 0.0036
81. 0.0175	82. 0.0830	

83. 18	84. 9	85. 1.08
86. 40	87. 25	88. 25%
89. 20%	90. 25%	91. 50
92. 120		

	Percent	Ratio	Common Fraction	Decimal
93.	25%	25 : 100	1/4	0.25
94.	3.3%	1 : 30	1/30	0.033
95.	5%	5 : 100	1/20	0.05
96.	0.67%	1 : 150	1/150	0.0067
97.	0.45%	45 : 100	9/20	0.0045
98.	1%	1 : 100	1/100	0.01
99.	0.83%	1 : 120	1/120	0.0083
100.	50%	50 : 100	1/2	0.50

CHAPTER 2: Common Fractions

Practice Problems: Pages 13–14

1. 7, 1/8, 7, 8   2. 9, 1/10, 10   3. 4, 1/5, 1, 5
4. 3, 1/4, 4

Practice Problems: Page 16

| 1. 1/2 | 2. 1/8 | 3. 1/9 |
| 4. 4/5 | 5. 4/6 | 6. 8/15 |

Order of size: smaller to larger value

1/300, 1/150, 1/100, 1/75, 1/25, 1/12, 1/9, 1/7, 1/3

Practice Problems: Page 20

1. 12/20	2. 20/40	3. 2/4
4. 5/8	5. 3/5	6. 6/10
7. 1/6	8. 1/6	9. 1/4
10. 1/18		

Practice Problems: Page 21

1. 1/6	2. 1/6	3. 1/9
4. 1/6	5. 1/9	6. 1/4
7. 1/3	8. 3/5	

Practice Problems: Page 25

1. 69/12	2. 55/8	3. 43/5
4. 136/9	5. 98/3	6. 87/4
7. 37/2	8. 57/9	9. 27/5
10. 67/6		

Practice Problems: Pages 26–27

1. 7 1/2	2. 6 5/6	3. 7 5/9
4. 6 6/11	5. 7 1/2	6. 2 2/3
7. 4 3/10	8. 7 3/4	9. 9 5/9
10. 18 2/3		

Practice Problems: Pages 37–38

1. 2 5/11	2. 13/16	3. 3 19/24
4. 1 2/45	5. 1 3/10	6. 1 9/19
7. 1 3/14	8. 10 23/45	9. 1 15/24
10. 1 17/30	11. 3/7	12. 4/9

13. 13/30   14. 19/36   15. 5 16/21
16. 1 1/12

Practice Problems: Page 43

1. 14/45	2. 5/21	3. 3/20
4. 1 7/20	5. 21/32	6. 40/77
7. 6 3/4	8. 1 2/13	9. 1 5/9
10. 36	11. 29/50	12. 3 5/7

End of Chapter Review: Pages 44–45

1. 14/35, 15/35	2. 28/20, 4/20	3. 1/6
4. 1/8	5. 6 1/2	6. 13 1/8
7. 50/11	8. 209/23	9. 5/16
10. 1/8	11. 1/9	12. 5/28
13. 8/9	14. 1 1/3	15. 31/36
16. 7 5/24	17. 1/6	18. 5/9
19. 7/12	20. 4 9/40	21. 2 1/8
22. 2 4/7	23. 3/20	24. 3/11
25. 14	26. 8	27. 6/11
28. 10	29. 1 5/7	30. 24
31. 10 4/15	32. 5/56	33. 80
34. 4 1/2		

CHAPTER 3: Decimal Fractions and Decimal Whole Numbers

Practice Problems: Pages 49–50

1. ten and one thousandths
2. three and seven ten-thousandths
3. eighty-three thousandths
4. one hundred and fifty-three thousandths
5. thirty-six and sixty-seven ten-thousandths

6. one hundred and twenty-five ten-thousandths
7. one hundred twenty-five and twenty-five thousandths
8. twenty and seventy-five thousandths

9. 5.037   10. 64.07   11. 0.020
12. 0.4   13. 8.064   14. 33.7
15. 0.015   16. 0.1

Practice Problems: Page 51

1. 0.75   2. 0.92   3. 1.75
4. 2.80

Practice Problems: Pages 59–60*

1. 38.2   2. 18.41   3. 84.64
4. 1.91   5. 19.91   6. 26.15
7. 243.58   8. 51.06   9. 12.33
10. 6.68   11. 66.25   12. 1.12
13. 22.51   14. 6.81   15. 101.4
16. 1065   17. 41.90   18. 7.94
19. 144.03   20. 400.14   21. 708.89
22. 30.54   23. 0.098   24. 0.0008
25. 9.32   26. 2.65   27. 10.89
28. 12.85

Practice Problems: Page 63*

1. 0.20   2. 0.125   3. 0.25
4. 0.067   5. 0.067   6. 0.053
7. 7/1,000   8. 93/100   9. 103/250
10. 5 3/100   11. 12 1/5   12. 1/8

*See Appendix B (pp. 333–334): Answers have been rounded off.

End of Chapter Review: Pages 64–65*

1. five and four hundredths
2. ten and sixty-five hundredths
3. eight thousandths
4. eighteen and nine tenths

5. 6.08	6. 124.3	7. 16.001
8. 24.45	9. 59.262	10. 2.776
11. 5.21	12. 224.52	13. 0.128
14. 1.56	15. 5.35	16. 16.2
17. 6.77	18. 4.26	19. 8.47
20. 3,387.58	21. 0.77	22. 981.67
23. 0.33	24. 0.60	25. 0.143
26. 0.75	27. 9/20	28. 3/4
29. 3/50	30. 0.40	31. 0.22
32. 0.80	33. 6 4/5	34. 1 7/20
35. 8 1/2		

CHAPTER 4: Percent, Ratio, and Proportion

Practice Problems: Page 71

1. 3/20	2. 3/10	3. 1/2
4. 3/4	5. 1/4	6. 3/5
7. 33 1/3%	8. 66.6%	9. 20%
10. 75%	11. 40%	12. 25%

Practice Problems: Page 75

1. 0.15	2. 0.25	3. 0.59
4. 0.80	5. 25%	6. 45%
7. 60%	8. 85%	9. 1/6 = 16.6%
10. 1/8 = 12.5%	11. 1/5 = 20%	12. 1/3 = 33.3%

*See Appendix B (pp. 333–334): Answers have been rounded off.

Practice Problems: Pages 85–86

1. $\dfrac{50 \text{ mg}}{5 \text{ mL}}$; 50 mg : 5 mL; 50 mg/5 mL

2. $\dfrac{325 \text{ mg}}{1 \text{ tablet}}$; 325 mg : 1 tab; 325 mg/1 tab

3. $\dfrac{2 \text{ ampules}}{1 \text{ liter}}$; 2 amps : 1 L; 2 amps/1 L

4. 250 mg/1 capsule; 250 mg : 1 capsule; 250 mg/capsule

5. $\dfrac{1 \text{ tablet}}{5 \text{ grains}} : \dfrac{3 \text{ tablets}}{15 \text{ grains}}$
   1 tab : 5 gr :: 3 tabs : 15 gr

6. $\dfrac{0.2 \text{ mg}}{1 \text{ tablet}} :: \dfrac{0.4 \text{ mg}}{2 \text{ tablets}}$
   0.2 mg : 1 tab :: 0.4 mg : 2 tabs

7. $\dfrac{10 \text{ mg}}{5 \text{ mL}} :: \dfrac{30 \text{ mg}}{15 \text{ mL}}$
   10 mg : 5mL :: 30 mg : 15 mL

8. $x = 9$

9. $x = 18$

10. $x = 4$

11. $x = 50$

12. $\dfrac{50 \text{ mg}}{1 \text{ mL}} = \dfrac{40}{x \text{ mL}}$
    $50x = 40 \qquad x = 0.8 \text{ mL}$

13. $\dfrac{25 \text{ mg}}{1 \text{ mL}} = \dfrac{x \text{ mg}}{1.5 \text{ mL}}$
    $x = 25 \times 1.5 \qquad x = 37.5 \text{ mg}$

14. $\dfrac{0.125 \text{ mg}}{1 \text{ tablet}} = \dfrac{x}{2 \text{ tablets}}$
    $x = 0.125 \times 2 \qquad x = 0.25 \text{ mg}$

15. 1 g/5 mL = x g/15 mL
    $5x = 15$ $x = 3$ g

End of Chapter Review: Pages 87–91

	Percent	Fraction	Decimal
1.	16.6%	1/6	0.166
2.	25%	1/4	0.25
3.	6.4%	8/125	0.064
4.	21%	21/100	0.21
5.	40%	2/5	0.40
6.	162%	1 31/50	1.62
7.	27%	27/100	0.27
8.	5 1/4%	21/400	0.052
9.	450%	9/2	4.50
10.	8 1/3%	1/12	0.083
11.	1%	1/100	0.01
12.	85.7%	6/7	0.857
13.	450%	18/4	4.5
14.	150%	1 1/2	1.5
15.	72%	18/25	0.72

16. $\dfrac{10 \text{ mg}}{1 \text{ tab}}$; 10 mg : 1 tab

17. $\dfrac{10 \text{ units}}{1 \text{ mL}}$; 10 units : 1 mL

18. $\dfrac{200 \text{ mg}}{1 \text{ kg}}$; 200 mg : kg

19. $\dfrac{100 \text{ mg}}{1 \text{ tab}} :: \dfrac{300 \text{ mg}}{x \text{ tab}}$
    100 mg : 1 tab :: 300 mg : x tab

20. $\dfrac{250 \text{ mg}}{1 \text{ tab}} :: \dfrac{500 \text{ mg}}{x \text{ tab}}$
    250 mg : 1 tab :: 500 mg : x tab

21. $\dfrac{0.075 \text{ mg}}{1 \text{ tab}} :: \dfrac{0.15 \text{ mg}}{x \text{ tab}}$

    0.075 mg : 1 tab :: 0.15 mg : x tab

22. 250 mg/0.5 mL :: 500 mg/x mL

    250 mg : 0.5 mL :: 500 mg : x mL

23. $\dfrac{4}{5}$ or 0.8

24. 6

25. 4.5

26. $x = 6$

27. 20 mg : 1 mL :: 10 mg : x mL

    20 mg $\times$ x mL = 10 mg $\times$ 1 mL

    $20x = 10$

    $\dfrac{\cancel{20}^{1}\, x}{\cancel{20}_{1}} = \dfrac{\cancel{10}^{1}}{\cancel{20}_{2}} = \dfrac{1}{2}\, x = \dfrac{1}{2}$ mL

    Answer: $\dfrac{1}{2}$ mL

    Verify the Answer:

    $\overbrace{20 \text{ mg} : 1 \text{ mL} :: 10 \text{ mg} : \underbrace{\dfrac{1}{2}\, (0.5) \text{ mL}}_{}}^{\text{EXTREMES}}$

    $\underbrace{\phantom{20 \text{ mg} : 1 \text{ mL} :: 10 \text{ mg}}}_{\text{MEANS}}$

    20 mg $\times$ 0.5 mL = 10 mg $\times$ 1 mL

    $\left.\begin{array}{l} 20 \times 0.5 = 10 \\ 10 \times 1 = 10 \end{array}\right\}$ Sum products are equal

    CTC* = Yes

28. $\dfrac{50 \text{ mg}}{5 \text{ mL}} = \dfrac{25 \text{ mg}}{x \text{ mL}}$

*CTC = Critical Thinking Check

Cross-multiply:

50 mg $\times$ x mL = 25 mg $\times$ 5 mL
50x = 125

$$\frac{\cancel{50}^{1}x}{\cancel{50}_{1}} = \frac{\cancel{125}^{5}}{\cancel{50}_{2}}$$

$$x = \frac{5}{2} = 2\frac{1}{2} \text{ mL}$$

Answer: 2.5 mL

Verify the Answer:

$$\frac{50 \text{ mg}}{5 \text{ mL}} = \frac{25 \text{ mg}}{2.5 \text{ mL}}$$

$$\left.\begin{array}{l} 50 \times 2.5 = 125 \\ 25 \times 5 = 125 \end{array}\right\} \begin{array}{l} \text{Sum products} \\ \text{are equal} \end{array}$$

CTC = Yes

29. 3.0 mg : 1.0 mL :: 1.5 mg : x mL
    3.0 mg $\times$ x mL = 1.5 mg $\times$ 1.0 mL
    3x = 1.5

$$\frac{\cancel{3}^{1}x}{\cancel{3}_{1}} = \frac{\cancel{1.5}^{1}}{\cancel{3}_{2}} = \frac{1}{2}$$

$$x = \frac{1}{2} \text{ mL}$$

Answer: $\frac{1}{2}$ mL

Verify the Answer:

$$\overbrace{3.0 \text{ mg} : \underbrace{1.0 \text{ mL} :: 1.5 \text{ mg}}_{\text{MEANS}} : 0.5 \text{ mL}}^{\text{EXTREMES}}$$

3.0 mg $\times$ 0.5 mL = 1.5 mg $\times$ 1.0 mL

$\left.\begin{array}{l} 3.0 \times 0.5 = 1.5 \\ 1.5 \times 1.0 = 1.5 \end{array}\right\}$ Sum products are equal

CTC = Yes

30. 20 mg : 2 mL :: 25 mg : x mL

20 mg $\times$ x mL = 25 mg $\times$ 2 mL

$20x = 50$

$\dfrac{\cancel{20}^{1}\, x}{\cancel{20}_{1}} = \dfrac{50}{20} = \dfrac{5}{2}\, x = 2.5$ mL

Answer: 2.5 mL

Verify the Answer:

20 mg : 2 mL :: 25 mg : 2.5 mL

20 mg $\times$ 2.5 mL = 25 mg $\times$ 2 mL

$\left.\begin{array}{l} 20 \times 2.5 = 50 \\ 25 \times 2 = 50 \end{array}\right\}$ Sum products are equal

CTC = Yes

31. 7.5 mL
32. 7.5 mL
33. 0.5 mL
34. 1.5 mL
35. 1.6 mL
36. 0.7 mL
37. 3 tablets

End of Unit 1 Review: Pages 92–94

1. 1	2. 1/15
3. 7/10	4. 5/12
5. 4/15	6. 1/16
7. 1/75	8. 1/150
9. 2	10. 4/5

11. 1/4
12. 3 1/3
13. 1/3
14. 1/6
15. 1/100
16. 5/30
17. 3.1
18. 4.26
19. 0.4
20. 5.68
21. 2.5
22. 15
23. 16.67
24. 1.89
25. 0.8
26. 0.25
27. 0.33
28. 1/2
29. 7/100
30. 1 1/2
31. 1/4
32. 1/300
33. 3/500
34. 40%
35. 450%
36. 2%
37. 12 (4 × 12 & 3 × 16 = 48)
38. 1 1/5 (25 × 1.2 & 20 × 1.5 = 30)
39. 1 1/4 (8 × 1.2 & 1 × 10 = 10)
40. 1 3/5 (4/5 × 50 & 25 × 1.6 = 40)
41. 1/2 (500 × 1/2 & 1,000 × 1/4 = 250)
42. 0.5 (100 × 1/2 & 2 × 2.5 = 50)
43. 180
44. 2
45. 1/9
46. 600
47. 1 3/5
48. 5
49. 10
50. 30
51. 1
52. 1/4
53. 1.25
54. 2
55. 1 1/3

CHAPTER 5: The Metric System

Practice Problems: Page 101

1. 0.036 m
2. 41.6 dm
3. 0.08 cm
4. 0.002 m
5. 2.05 cm
6. 180 mm
7. 3,000 mm
8. 0.02 m

Practice Problems: Page 104

1. 0.0036 L	2. 61.7 mL
3. 900 mL	4. 64 mg
5. 1.0 g	6. 0.008 dg

End of Chapter Review: Pages 105–106

1. 0.00743 m	2. 0.006 dm
3. 10,000 m	4. 6217 mm
5. 0.0164 dL	6. 0.047 L
7. 1,000 cL	8. 569 mL
9. 0.0356 g	10. 30 cg
11. 50 mg	12. 930 mg
13. 0.1 mg	14. 2,000 mcg
15. 0.001 mg	16. 7,000 g
17. 4,000 mcg	18. 13,000 g
19. 2,500 mL	20. 600 mcg
21. 80 mg	22. 10 mcg
23. 0.06 g	24. 10,500 mcg
25. 0.0005 L	26. 1 dg
27. 3.5 g	28. 0.0034 g
29. 3,000 mcg	30. 0.13 g
31. 2,000 g	32. 18,000 mL
33. 450,000 mg	34. 0.04 mg
35. 8,000 dL	36. 100 cL
37. 460 dg	38. 500 mg
39. 5 L	40. 0.025 g

CHAPTER 6: The Apothecary System and Household Measurements

End of Chapter Review: Pages 118–119

1. gr iii	2. ℥ v	3. f℥ vii
4. mx	5. mxxss̄	6. pt v

7. 2   8. 960 m   9. 32
10. 1/2   11. 1   12. 2
13. 1/4 pt   14. ℥ 1/4   15. ℥ ii
16. ℥ iv   17. 2 cups   18. 24 oz
19. 3 oz   20. 120 gtt   21. 9 tsp
22. 12 oz   23. 1/2 pt   24. 1 pt
25. 4 T   26. 2 oz   27. 6 oz
28. 1.5 qt   29. 1 oz   30. 32 oz
31. 30 gtt

CHAPTER 7: Approximate Equivalents and System Conversions

Practice Problems: Pages 125–126

1. 48–60 mL   2. 0.0003 L   3. 45–48 m
4. 0.75 gr   5. 8–10 mL   6. 66 lbs
7. 0.3 mg   8. 1,500 mL   9. 24–30 g
10. 0.3 mg   11. 1 oz   12. 60 mL
13. gr 1/10   14. 45 gr   15. 1 quart
16. 2 L   17. 1 Kg   18. ℥ iv

End of Chapter Review: Pages 127–129

1. 25 kg   2. 60 g
3. 960 mL/day   4. 4 inches
5. 1 tsp   6. 300–325 mg
7. 3 gtt   8. gr 1/150
9. ℥ viii   10. 300 mcg or 0.3 mg
11. 1.8 g   12. 2 oz
13. 6 tablets   14. 1 tsp; f℥ 1
15. 15 mL or 3 tsp   16. 0.4 gram
17. 125 mg; 1 g   18. 450 mL
19. 25 mL   20. 2 teaspoons
21. 0.5 mL   22. 2 tablets; 60 mg

End of Unit 2 Review: Pages 130-131

1. 80 mg	2. 3,200 mL
3. 1.5 mg	4. 125 mcg
5. 20,000 g	6. 0.005 g
7. 4 drams	8. ℥ss
9. 1/4	10. 16 ounces
11. 1 1/2 quarts	12. ℥ i
13. 3 teaspoons	14. 1 ounce
15. 6 ounces	16. 1 ounce
17. 30 mg	18. 1 ounce
19. 30 mL	20. 60–65 mg
21. 15 mL	22. 44 pounds
23. 0.4 mg	24. gr 1/200
25. 54 mL	26. 4 tsp
27. 8,500 mg	28. 0.9 g
29. 1/4 gr	30. 6,000

CHAPTER 8: Medication Labels

Practice Problems: Pages 141–143

FIGURE 8.2 (Requip)

1. Ropinirole hydrochloride
2. NDC 0007-4895-20
3. 3 mg
4. 100 tablets
5. Tablets
6. Protect from light and moisture. Close container tightly after each use.
7. Requip
8. GlaxoSmithKline

FIGURE 8.3 (Augmentin)

1. Amoxicillin/clavulanate potassium
2. 200 mg/5 mL

3. Keep tightly closed. Shake well before using. Must be refrigerated. Discard after 10 days.
4. Add 2/3 of total water for reconstitution.
5. Each 5 mL contains amoxicillin 200 mg.
6. 50 mL.

FIGURE 8.4 (Ancef)

1. Cefazolin
2. Intramuscular and intravenous
3. 2.5 mL of sterile water for injection
4. 330 mg/mL (IM use)
5. 250 mg to 1 gram, every 6–8 hours
6. Shake well. Before reconstitution, protect from light and store at 20–25 degrees Centrigrade (room temperature).

End of Chapter Review: Pages 144–146

FIGURES 8.5 to 8.9 (Tagamet, Amoxil, Augmentin, Paxil, Ancef)

1. 1 tablet; 1200 mg	2. 500 mg; 0.5 grams
3. 2.5 mL; 300 mg; 7.5 mL	4. 1 tablet; 80 mg
5. 1 vial	6. 2.5 mL

CHAPTER 9: Oral Dosage Calculations

Practice Problems: Pages 159–163

1. 4 tablets	2. 15 mL
3. 1/2 tablet	4. 10 mL
5. 3 tablets	6. 2 tablets
7. 5 mL	8. 1/2 tablet
9. 3/5 tablet	10. 4 tablets
11. 3 tablets	12. 12 mL
13. 15 mL	14. 10 mL

15. 2 tablets;
    CTC = No
16. 12.5 mL

17. 8 tablets
18. 8–10 mL;
    CTC = No

19. 3 tablets
20. 4 tablets

21. 2 tablets
22. 15 mL; 30 mg

23. 1/2 tsp; 7.5 mL
24. gr 1/60

25. 18.8 mL
26. 2 tablets

27. 2 tablets
28. 1 tablet

29. 2 tsp
30. 1 tablet

31. 10 mL; 2 tsp
32. 15 mL; 1/2 oz

33. 2 capsules

End of Chapter Review: Pages 164–166

 1. 3 tablets
 2. 3 tablets

 3. 30 mL
 4. 4 tablets

 5. 1 tablet
 6. 2 tablets

 7. 1 ounce
 8. 1 tablet

 9. 7.5 mL
10. 1 tablet

11. 1 tablet;
    4 tablets
12. 4 tablets;
    CTC = Yes

13. 4 tablets
14. 1 tsp; 2 i

15. 10 mL; 2 tsp;
    CTC = Yes
16. 50 mg

17. 4 tablets
18. 2 tablets

19. 1 tablet

CHAPTER 10: Parenteral Dosage Calculations

End of Chapter Review: Pages 179–183

1. 2 mL
2. 2 mL

3. 3 mL
4. 2 mL

5. 0.8 mL   6. 2.5 mL; CTC = Yes
7. 0.4 mL   8. 0.75 mL
9. 0.7 mL   10. 3 mL
11. 0.6 mL   12. 0.25 mL
13. 0.75 mL   14. 1.25 mL
15. 0.8 mL   16. 0.8 mL; CTC = No
17. 0.6 mL   18. 0.75 mL
19. 0.5 mL   20. 2.0 mL
21. 2 mL   22. 0.5 mL
23. 1.5 mL;   24. 1 mL
    CTC = No
25. 2 mL   26. 0.5 mL
27. 1.5 mL   28. 0.25 mL
29. 4 mL   30. 1 mL
31. 1.2 mL   32. 0.5 mL
33. 2.5 mL
34. 4 mL; CTC = No. Limit injection to 3 mL/site.

CHAPTER 11: Intravenous Therapies

Practice Problems: Pages 201–203

1. 83 mL/hr; CTC = Yes   2. 125 mL/hr
3. 27 gtt/min   4. 42 gtt/min
5. 21 gtt/min   6. 17 gtt/min; CTC =
                            slower @ 13 gtt/min
7. 17 gtt/min   8. 19 gtt/min
9. 20 gtt/min   10. 50 gtt/min
11. 19 gtt/min   12. 17 gtt/min
13. 25 mL; 25 gtt/min;   14. 67 gtt/min
    CTC = Yes

End of Chapter Review: Pages 204–206

1. 63 mL/hr   2. 100 mL/hr
3. 250 mL/hr   4. 83 mL/hr

5. 50 mL/hr
6. 63 mL/hr
7. 21 gtt/min
8. 42 gtt/min
9. 167 mL/hr;
28 gtt/min
10. 10 gtt/min
11. 19 gtt/min
12. 8 gtt/min
13. 20 hr
14. 12 1/2 hr
15. 12 1/2 hr
16. 13 gtt/min
17. 42 gtt/min
18. 38 gtt/min
19. 100 gtt/min
20. 125 mL
21. 3.0 mL
22. 10 gtt/min
23. 100 mL/hr; 34 gtt/min

CHAPTER 12: Intravenous Therapies: Critical-Care Applications

End of Chapter Review: Pages 219–222

1. 3 mL/hr; CTC 5 Yes
2. 4 mg/min
3. 15.1 mL/hr; CTC 5 decrease to 7.6 mL/hr
4. 22.2 mcg/kg/min
5. 3 mL/hr
6. 40 mL; 1 mg/mL; 60 mL/hr
7. 1 mL; 200 mL/hr; 15.1 mL/hr
8. 2 mL; 25 mL; 10 mL/hr
9. 7.22 mcg/kg/min; CTC 5 increases to 10.8 mcg/kg/min
10. 7.5 mL/min; 80 mcg/min
11. 10 mL/hr
12. 200 mcg/mL; 67–68 mL/hr
13. 10 mL; 6 mL/hr
14. 11.2 mL/hr; CTC = increase to 18.8 mL/hr; increase to 22.5 mL/hr
15. 6 mL/hr

16. 4 mcg/min
17. 10 mL/hr
18. 14 mL/hr

CHAPTER 13: Insulin

End of Chapter Review: Pages 233–236

1. 60 U of U-100

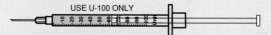

2. 82 U of U-100

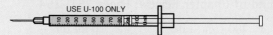

3. 45 U of U-100

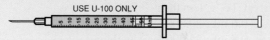

4. 35 U of U-100

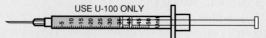

5. 26 U of U-100

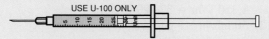

6. 56 U of U-100

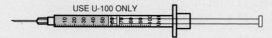

7. 60 U	8. 40 U
9. 20 U	10. 70 U
11. 21; U-30/0.5 mL	12. 45; U-50/0.5 mL
13. 64; U-100/1 mL	14. 38; U-50/0.5 mL
15. 30; U-30/0.5 mL	16. U-50; 30 U;
	CTC = Not Logical
17. 39 U; U-50	18. 15 U
19. 50 U; CTC = Logical	20. 34 U; NPH

CHAPTER 14: Heparin Preparation and Dosage Calculations

End of Chapter Review: Pages 251–254

1. 400 U/hr; safe
2. 20 mL/hr
3. 20 mL/hr; 20 gtt/min
4. 4,480 U; 20.2 mL/hr
5. 22.4 mL/hr;
   CTC = less than
6. 11.4 U/kg/hr
7. 0.6 mL; 20,000 U; is within
8. 0.8 mL; 24,000 U; is within;
   CTC = 15,000 U/8 hr
9. 0.6 mL; 10,000 U;
   is within
10. 0.25 mL
11. 600 U/hr
12. 1.5 mL/min = 90 mL/hr;
    1,350 U/hr = 32,400 U/24 hr
13. 50 mL/hr; 17 gtt/min
14. 21 mL/hr; 625 U/hr
15. 6 gtt/min
16. 12.7 mL/hr
17. 13.1 U/kg/hr

CHAPTER 15: Pediatric Dosage Calculations and Intravenous Therapy

Practice Problems: Pages 270–273

1. No; safe dosage range is 300 mg/day
2. Yes; safe dosage range is 100–200 mg/day
3. 4 mg; Yes; safe dosage range is 0.8–4 mg/dose
4. 11 mL
5. 50 kg; 50–70 mg/dose; No
6. 60 kg; 750–1,500 mg/dose; Yes
7. 30 kg; 187.5–375 mg/dose; Yes
8. 15 kg; 37.5–75 mg/dose; Yes
9. 20 kg; 5–20 mg/dose; 4 mL; Yes
10. 12.5–25 mg/dose; Yes
11. 12.5–50 mg/dose; Yes
12. 80–120 mg; 1 mL; Yes
13. 300 mg; 600 mg; Yes;
    CTC = No, 24-hour total = 900 mg
14. 1.5 mL
15. 300 mg; 3 mL

End of Chapter Review: Pages 278–284

1. 10 mg; is safe
2. 250 mg
3. 30 mg in 0.6 mL
4. 10 mg in 4 mL
5. 0.8 mg in 2 mL
6. 20 mg
7. 15 kg; 375–750 mg; 6 mL/q6h = 600 mg/day
   is safe
8. 30 kg; 90–150 mg/day; 100 mg; is safe;
   CTC = Yes, dosage = 100 mg

9. 7 mg; 1.4 mL
10. Surface area = 1.03 m²; Dosage = 30 mg dose
11. 0.8 mL
12. 0.5 mL
13. 650 mg/day; Yes; 6.5 mL
14. 125–250 mg/dose; Yes
15. Yes
16. 200–400 mg/dose; Yes
17. No
18. 7.5–24.75 mg/dose; Yes
19. 600–1,200 mg/dose; 1,000 mg; Yes
20. 2.5–10 mg/day; 0.5 mL; Yes
21. 0.6 mL; is safe
22. 40 kg; 2–8 mg; 0.33 mL; is safe
23. 30 kg; 1,200/day; 300 mg; is safe
24. 40 kg; 20–80 mg; 4 mL; is safe
25. 90 mL/hr
26. 130 mL/hr
27. 130 mL/hr
28. 93 mL/hr
29. 120 mL/hr
30. 75 mL/hr
31. 30 gtt/min
32. 60 gtt/min; 60 mL
33. 0.5 mL
34. 15 gtt/min

CHAPTER 16: Solutions

End of Chapter Review: Pages 294–295

1. 8 grams
2. 300 mL; 1,200 mL
3. 375 mL; 125 mL
4. 1.8 mL
5. 3 mL
6. 2 mL

End of Unit 3 Review: Pages 296–302

1. 6 tablets
2. 500 mg
3. 3 tablets
4. 5 mL
5. 15 mL; CTC = Yes, 15 mL = 1 tbsp
6. 1/2 tablet
7. 1 tablet
8. 2 mL
9. 1 mL
10. 3 mL
11. 30 mL
12. 0.5 mL
13. 1.5 mL
14. 1.25 mL
15. 1.66 mL
16. 3 mL
17. 3 mL
18. 200 mL
19. 21 gtt/min; CTC = greater at 32/min
20. 50 gtt/min (approximate)
21. 41.6 gtt/min (approximate)
22. 11 hours; 6 minutes
23. 5 mg/hr; 83 mcg/min
24. 15
25. 10 units of Regular; 35 units of NPH
26. 0.5 mL
27. 450 units/hr
28. 20 gtt/min
29. 1,000 units/hr is a safe dose
30. 0.5 mL/10 doses
31. Yes
32. 20–30 mg/dose; 0.5 mL; Yes
33. 10–34 mg/dose; 0.75 mL; Yes
34. 13–16.25 mg/dose; 1.5 mL; Yes
35. 400 mg/dose; 400 mg; Yes
36. 5–10 mg/dose; 0.4 mL; Yes
37. 0.1 mL
38. 0.5 mL
39. 12.4 grams
40. 16 mg

41. 1 tablet; 9 mg
42. 6 units/hr
43. 6 mg/hr
44. 3 mL/hr

Appendix B: Rounding Off Decimals

Practice Problems: Page 334

1. 0.8	2. 0.3
3. 0.2	4. 1.2
5. 2.7	6. 3.8

1. 0.55	2. 0.74
3. 1.68	4. 1.23
5. 2.47	6. 4.38

A

Roman Numerals

The use of Roman numerals dates back to ancient times when symbols were used for pharmaceutical computations and record keeping. Modern medicine still uses Roman numerals in prescribing medications, especially when using the apothecary system of weights and measurement.

The Roman system uses letters to designate numbers; the most commonly used letters can be found in Table A-1. Lowercase Roman numerals are used to express numbers. The most common letters you will use are 1/2 ($\overline{\text{ss}}$), one (i), five (v), and 10 (x). Four numerals are rarely used in practice (50, 100, 500, 1,000) but are included in the table.

The Roman numeral system follows certain rules for arrangement of its numerals.

> ● **RULE: To read and write Roman numerals, follow these steps:**

TABLE A.1 Roman Numeral Equivalents for Arabic Numerals

ARABIC NUMERAL	ROMAN NUMERAL
1/2	$\overline{ss}$
1	i
2	ii
3	iii
4	iv
5	v
6	vi
7	vii
8	viii
9	ix
10	x
15	xv
20	xx
30	xxx
50	L
100	C
500	D
1,000	M

- Add values when the *largest* valued numeral is on the *left* and the *smallest* valued numeral is on the *right*.

Examples: xv = 10 + 5 = 15

xxv = 20 + 5 = 25

- Subtract values when the *smallest* valued numeral is on the *left* and the *largest* valued numeral is on the *right*.

Examples: ix = 1 − 10 = 9
iv = 1 − 5 = 4

- *Subtract* values *first* and then *add* when the *smallest* valued numeral is in the *middle* and the *larger* values are on either side.

Examples: xiv = (1 − 5) = 4 + 10 = 14
xix = (1 − 10) = 9 + 10 = 19

> ● **RULE: To repeat Roman numerals, follow this step:**

- Roman numerals of the same value can be repeated in sequence, *only up to three times*. Once you can no longer repeat, you need to subtract.

Examples: 3 = iii
4 = 5 (v) − 1 (i) = iv
9 = 10 (x) − 1 (i) = ix
30 = 10 (x) + 10 (x) + 10 (x) = xxx
40 = 50 (L) − 10 (X) = XL

Note: Three numerals *may never be repeated* in sequence because their values, when doubled, become separate Roman numerals. These are L, V, and D.

Examples: X = 10   not   VV
C = 100   not   LL
M = 1,000   not   DD

Note: You can only add and subtract in the Roman numeral system.

Rounding Off Decimals

To round off decimals, follow these steps:

- Determine the place that the decimal is to be "rounded off" to (tenths, hundredths). For example, let's round off 36.315 to the nearest hundredth.
- Bracket the number [ ] in the hundredths place (2 places to the right of the decimal). For 36.315, you would bracket the 1. Then 36.315 would look like this: 36.3[1]5.
- Look at the number to the right of the bracket. For 36.3[1]5, that number would be 5.
- If the number to the right of the bracket is less than 5 (<5), then drop the number. If it is 5 or greater than 5 (>5), then increase the bracketed number by 1.

For 36.3[1]5, increase the bracketed number [1] by 1.
The rounded off number becomes 36.32.

Example: 5.671
5.6[7]1
Look at the number to the right of [7].
The number is <5.
Leave [7] as is; drop 1.
[7] stays as [7].
5.671 rounds off to 5.67.

Answer: 5.67

PRACTICE PROBLEMS

Round off to the nearest tenth.

1. 0.83 _____   2. 0.34 _____

3. 0.19 _____   4. 1.19 _____

5. 2.66 _____   6. 3.84 _____

Round off to the nearest hundredth.

1. 0.545 _____   2. 0.737 _____

3. 1.680 _____   4. 1.231 _____

5. 2.468 _____   6. 4.383 _____

Answers are on p. 328.

C

Abbreviations and Symbols for Drug Preparation and Administration

ABBREVIATION/SYMBOL	INTERPRETATION
a or ā	before
@	at
aa or āā	of each
a.c.	before meals
A.D.	right ear
ad lib.	as desired
A.L. or A.S.	left ear
alt. h.	alternate hour
AM	before noon
aq.	water

ABBREVIATION/SYMBOL	INTERPRETATION
A.S.A.P.	as soon as possible
A.U.	both ears
b.i.d.	twice a day
b.i.n.	twice a night
b.i.w.	twice a week
$\bar{c}$	with
C	gallon
cap(s).	capsule(s)
cc	cubic centimeter
CD	controlled dose
cm	centimeter
CR	controlled release
D/C	discontinue
DS	double strength
dil.	dilute
disp.	dispense
dr or ʒ	dram
Dx	diagnose
elix.	elixir
ext.	extract; external
fl; fld	fluid
g	gram
gal	gallon
gr	grain
gtt	drops
h, hr	hour
Ⓗ	hypodermic
h.s.	hour of sleep; at bedtime
ID	intradermal
IM	intramuscular
IN	intranasal
IV	intravenous
IVPB	intravenous piggyback
kg	kilogram
KVO	keep vein open
L	liter
LA	long acting
lb	pound

ABBREVIATION/SYMBOL	INTERPRETATION
M; m	meter
m; min	minim
mcg	microgram
mEq	milliequivalent
mg	milligram
mL	milliliter
mm	millimeter
NGT	narogastric tube
noct., NOC	at night
N.P.O.	nothing by mouth
NSS, NS	normal saline solution
O.	pint
O.D.	right eye
o.d.; q.d.	once every day
o.h.	every hour
oint	ointment
o.m.	every morning
o.n.	every night
O.S.	left eye
OTC	over-the-counter
O.U.	both eyes
oz	ounce
$\bar{p}$	after
p.c.	after meals
per	by
p.o. or per os	by mouth
PM	evening, before midnight
p.r.n.	as needed; when necessary
PSS	physiologic saline solution
pt	pint
q*	each; every
q.a.m	every morning
qh	every hour
q.i.d.	four times a day
q2h	every 2 hours
q3h	every 3 hours

*Some hospitals now require that the word "every" be used instead of "q" to try to reduce the number of medication errors.

ABBREVIATION/SYMBOL	INTERPRETATION
q4h	every 4 hours
q6h	every 6 hours
q8h	every 8 hours
q12h	every 12 hours
q.o.d.	every other day
q.s.	quantity sufficient; as much as needed
qt	quart
R, rect	rectally
R_x	to take; by prescription
R/O	rule out
$\overline{s}$	without
$\overline{ss}$	one-half
SC, s.c.; s.q., sub q	subcutaneously
sig.	label; write
SL; subl.	sublingual
sol; soln	solution
s.o.s.	one dose as necessary
SR	sustained release
stat.	immediately
supp.	suppository
susp.	suspension
tab	tablet
tbs; T	tablespoon
t.i.d.	three times a day
tinct; tr	tincture
T.K.O.	to keep open
tsp; t	teaspoon
μg	microgram
ung.	ointment
vag.	vaginally
XL	long acting
XR	extended release

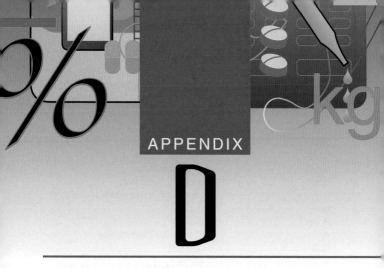

D

Intradermal Injections

The *intradermal route* is preferred for:

- Small quantities of medication (0.1 mL–0.2 mL)
- Nonirritating solutions that are slowly absorbed
- Allergy testing
- PPD administration (screening for tuberculosis)

The Intradermal Route
Use
A tuberculin syringe
Inject
Into dermis or upper layer of tissue under the outer layer of skin or epidermis. Make sure the bevel of the needle is up.
Angle
15 degrees   15°

Administering an Intradermal Injection

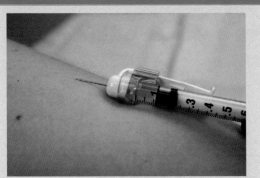

Inserting the needle almost level with the skin. (From Taylor, C., Lillis, C., LeMone, P., and Lynn, P. [2008]. *Fundamentals of nursing: The art and science of nursing care.* [6th ed.] Philadelphia: Lippincott Williams & Wilkins, p. 834.)

Gauge		Needle Length		Solution	
Range	*Average*	*Range*	*Average*	*Range*	*Average*
27–25	26	$\frac{3}{8} - \frac{5}{8}$	$\frac{1}{2}$	0.1 mL– 0.5mL	0.1 mL

Subcutaneous Injections

The Subcutaneous Route

Use
- An insulin syringe
- A prefilled disposable syringe with appropriate needle length

Inject
Under the skin into the fibrous tissue above the muscle

Angle*
45–90 degrees

45°   90°

*A 45-degree angle of insertion is used with a 5/8" needle for subcutaneous medications *except insulin and heparin,* for example, codeine sulfate and oxy-morphone hydrochloride. A 90-degree angle of insertion is used with a 3/8" to 1/2" needle for *insulin and heparin.*

Administering a Subcutaneous Injection

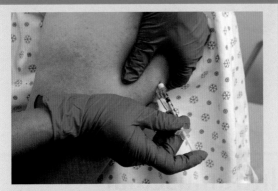

Bunching tissue around injection site. (From Taylor, C., Lillis, C., LeMone, P., and Lynn, P. [2008]. *Fundamentals of nursing: The art and science of nursing care* [6th ed.]. Philadelphia: Lippincott Williams & Wilkins, p. 837.)

Gauge		Needle Length		Solution	
Range	*Average*	*Range*	*Average*	*Range*	*Average*
27–25	26	$\dfrac{3}{8} - \dfrac{5}{8}$	$\dfrac{3}{8} - \dfrac{1}{2}$ c̄ 90° $\dfrac{5}{8}$ c̄ 45°	0.2 mL–2.0 mL	<0.1 mL

F

Intramuscular Injections

The *intramuscular route* is preferred for medications that:

- Are irritating to subcutaneous tissue
- Require a rapid rate of absorption
- Can be administered in volumes up to 5.0 mL

The Intramuscular Route

Use
A 3.0-mL to 5.0-mL syringe

Inject
Into the body of a striated muscle. Inject past the dermis and subcutaneous tissue. Always aspirate before injecting.

Angle
Always 90 degrees

▼ 90°

Administering an Intramuscular Injection

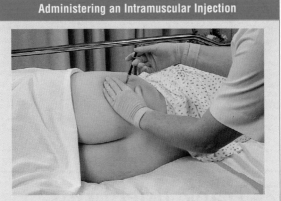

Spreading the skin at site and injecting medication at 90-degree angle. (From Taylor, C., Lillis, C., and LeMone, P. [2001]. *Fundamentals of nursing: The art and science of nursing care* [4th ed.]. Philadelphia: Lippincott Williams & Wilkins, p. 607.)

Gauge		Needle Length		Solution	
Range	*Average*	*Range*	*Average*	*Range*	*Average*
25–20	22	0.1–2.0 in.	1.5 in.	0.5 mL–5.0 mL	1.0 mL

Z-Track Injections

The *Z-track* method is used for parenteral drug administration when tissue damage from the leakage of irritating medications is expected or when it is essential that all of the medication can be absorbed in the muscle and not in the subcutaneous tissue. The method is easy, popular, and recommended by some institutions as a safe way of administering all intra-muscular injections. This method prevents "tracking" of the medication along the path of the needle during insertion and removal.

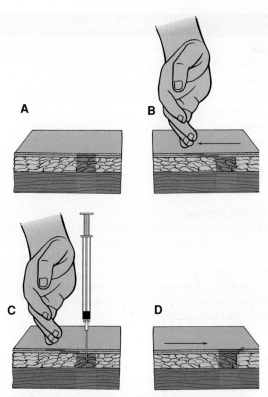

The Z-track or zigzag technique is recommended for intramuscular injections. **(A)** Normal skin and tissues. **(B)** Moving the skin to one side. **(C)** Needle is inserted at a 90-degree angle, and the nurse aspirates for blood. **(D)** Once the needle is withdrawn, displaced tissue is allowed to return to its normal position, preventing the solution from escaping from the muscle tissue. (From Taylor, C., Lillis, C., LeMone, P., and Lynn, P. [2008]. *Fundamentals of nursing: The art and science of nursing care* [6th ed.]. Philadelphia: Lippincott Williams & Wilkins, p. 840.)

The *Z*-Track Route

Use
A 3.0- to 5.0-mL syringe

Inject
Deep into the body of the gluteal muscle; the vastus lateralis can also be used.

Angle
Always 90 degrees

↓ 90°

Injection Technique
Displace or push tissue over muscle toward the center of the body by displacing the tissue with the last three fingers of the nondominant hand. Hold the tissues in this displaced position before, during, and for 5 to 15 seconds after the injection so the medication can begin to be absorbed. Use the IM injection technique as described in Appendix F.

Pediatric Intramuscular Injections

The Intramuscular Route

Use

A needle about 1" in length. For infants a 5/8" needle may be used.

Inject

Into dense muscle mass in the deltoid and ventrogluteal muscles. Into the outer quadrant of the gluteal and vastus lateralis muscles.

Angle

Preferably 45 degrees. May use 90 degrees if child's age and body mass warrant it.

The Intramuscular Route (continued)

Injection Technique

Similar to the intramuscular technique for adults as described on pages 343–344.

Gauge		Needle Length		Solution	
Range	*Average*	*Range*	*Average*	*Range*	*Average*
22–20	22	0.5 in–1.5 in	1.0 in	0.5 mL–2.5 mL	0.5–1.0 <3 yrs 0.5–1.5 4–6 yrs 0.5–2.0 7–14 yrs 1.0–2.5 >15 yrs

Nursing Concerns for Pediatric Drug Administration

When administering medications to children, you need to be aware of the following:

- Explain honestly what will be done; explain at the level of the child's understanding.
- Use supplemental materials to promote understanding (stuffed animals, dolls).
- Suggest that the child help as much as possible; encourage the child to pretend and switch roles with the child.
- Reinforce positive behavior with praise and rewards if necessary.
- Make sure you have obtained an accurate height and weight measurement.

- Be sure that you have compared the normal dose range with the dosage you plan to give; know toxic and lethal doses.
- Do not force medication on a frightened child, especially one who is crying.
- Always use two people when giving injections to small children.
- Disguise or dilute medications if necessary.

A nurse also needs to understand that the child's immature body system may respond differently to drugs, so there may be changes in an agent's absorption, distribution, biotransformation, and elimination. (See Appendix H for information about pediatric intramuscular injections.)

Nursing Considerations for Critical-Care Drug Administration

A patient who is critically ill may experience rapid hemodynamic changes. The nurse must possess knowledge of the medications administered and the effect of these medications on vital signs. Therefore, the nurse needs to be aware of the following considerations when administering medications to a patient who is critically ill:

- Blood pressure, pulse, and heart rhythms must be monitored frequently to titrate medications based on prescribed parameters.

- Drugs may be given to increase blood pressure (vasopressors) or to decrease blood pressure (vasodilators).
- Calculation of drug dosages and flow rates, which can be complicated, may need to be checked by another nurse or the pharmacist.
- Intravenous medications must be monitored carefully because their effects are immediate.
- The patient must be monitored closely for adverse drug reactions because critical-care medications have potent effects.
- Drugs are commonly started at a low dose and titrated to achieve the desired effect.
- Intravenous insertion sites must be monitored closely for signs of infiltration. Some vasopressors, such as dopamine, can cause tissue necrosis.
- Critical-care patients commonly have multiple drug infusions running at the same time. The nurse must check drug compatibilities before administering two medications together in the same intravenous site.

K

Nursing Concerns for Geriatric Drug Administration

As with pediatric medications, special consideration is given when administering drugs to anyone who is over 65 years. This is because physiologic changes caused by aging change the way the body reacts to certain drugs. For example, a tranquilizer may increase restlessness and agitation in an elderly person.

You should be aware of the following general considerations before administering a drug to any elderly individual.

- Small, frail elderly individuals will probably require less than the normal adult dosages. Drug absorption and distribution are affected by decreased gastrointestinal motility, decreased muscle mass, and diminished tissue perfusion.

- A drug should be given orally rather than parenterally, if possible, because decreased activity in the elderly decreases muscle tissue absorption.
- Often, it will be necessary to crush pills, empty capsules, or dissolve medications in liquid in order to assist the person to swallow without discomfort. Tell the patient *not to crush* enteric-coated or time-released drugs.
- Sedatives and narcotics must be given with extreme caution to elderly people, for they may easily become oversedated.
- Because the elderly are often on many different medications, you should check for drug interactions that may cause hazardous effects (e.g., giving a sedative shortly after a tranquilizer).
- The cumulative side effects of the drugs being administered must be monitored. A drug's excretion may be altered if the patient has reduced renal blood flow and reduced kidney function.
- A schedule for rotation of injection sites should be followed carefully because the elderly have decreased muscle mass and increased vascular fragility.
- Any written directions for medication administration should be clear and in large print because of possible impaired vision.
- The problem of impaired hearing should be remembered when giving directions or asking questions. You may have to speak very loudly or repeat the same information several times.

Writing the directions is recommended for some patients.
- Reinforce any important information by asking the patient to repeat it for you. This also helps you to ascertain whether the information was understood. Memory loss and confusion are common in the elderly because of cerebral arteriosclerosis.

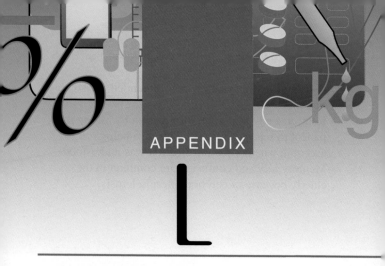

APPENDIX

L

Needleless
Intravenous
System

Shown on page 357 are a syringe prepared to inject
into needleless port and a piggyback setup connected
to a needleless port. (Photo by Rick Brady.) (From
Taylor, C., Lillis, C., and LeMone, P. [2008].
*Fundamentals of nursing: The art and science of
nursing care* [6th ed.]. Philadelphia: Lippincott
Williams & Wilkins, pp. 792 and 851.)

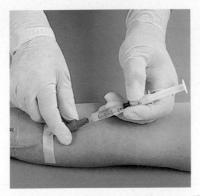

Syringe prepared to inject into needleless port. (From Taylor, C., Lillis, C., LeMone, P., and Lynn, P. [2008]. *Fundamentals of nursing: The art and science of nursing care* [6th ed.]. Philadelphia: Lippincott Williams & Wilkins, p. 792.)

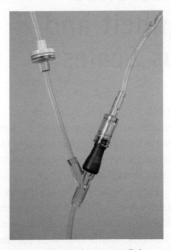

Piggyback setup connected to a needleless port. (From Taylor, C., Lillis, C., LeMone, P., and Lynn, P. [2008]. *Fundamentals of nursing: The art and science of nursing care* [6th ed.]. Philadelphia: Lippincott Williams & Wilkins, p. 851.)

Temperature Conversions: Fahrenheit and Celsius Scales

Electronic digital thermometers, which convert between the scales, are popular today. However, it is still necessary for health care practitioners to understand the differences between the scales and to be able to apply the conversion formulas.

The differences between the scales, as shown below, are based on the differences between the boiling and freezing points. This difference, 180 (F) and 100 (C), forms the basis for the conversion formulas.

Scale	Abbreviation	Boiling Point	Freezing Point
Fahrenheit	F	212	32
Centigrade	C	100	0

RULE: To change from Fahrenheit to Celsius, perform the following steps:

- Subtract 32 degrees from the Fahrenheit reading.
- Divide by 9/5 (1.8) or, for convenience, multiply by 5/9.
- $C = (F - 32) \times \dfrac{5}{9}$

Example: Convert 100°F to Celsius.

$$\begin{array}{c} 100 \\ -\ 32 \\ \hline 68 \end{array} \qquad \frac{68}{1} \times \frac{5}{9} = \frac{340}{9}$$

$$= 340 \div 9 = 37.7°C$$

Answer: 37.7° Celsius

RULE: To change from Celsius to Fahrenheit, perform the following steps:

- Multiply the Celsius reading by 9/5 or 1.8.
- Add 32.
- $F = (9/5 \times C \text{ or } C \times 1.8) + 32$

Example: Convert 40°C to Fahrenheit.

$$40^{\,8} \times \frac{9}{5_{\,1}} = 72$$

or

$$40 \times 1.8 = 72$$

$$\begin{array}{r} 72 \\ +32 \\ \hline 104° \end{array}$$

Answer: 104° Fahrenheit

You may find the following temperature conversion scale useful for quick reference.

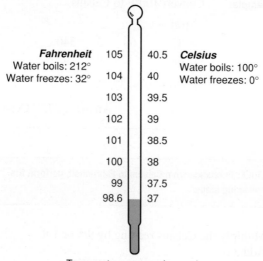

Fahrenheit	105	40.5	*Celsius*
Water boils: 212°	104	40	Water boils: 100°
Water freezes: 32°	103	39.5	Water freezes: 0°
	102	39	
	101	38.5	
	100	38	
	99	37.5	
	98.6	37	

Temperature conversion scale

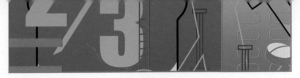

Index

Page numbers followed by *app* indicate appendices; page numbers followed by *f* indicate figures; and *t* following a page number indicates tabular material.